Dr. Alan H. Pressman, D.C., Ph.D., D.A.C.B.N., C.C.N., is a chiropractor and a board certified dietitian/nutritionist. He is the former chairman of the Department of Clinical Nutrition at New York Chiropractic College and served numerous terms as president for the Council on Nutrition of the American Chiropractic Association. He is also a diplomate and past president of the American Chiropractic Board of Nutrition.

Dr. Pressman has been a regular contributor on CNBC and is a noted veteran radio guest on ABC and WOR talk radio. His expertise on a wide range of topical health issues has been heard by millions on the nationally syndicated radio show, *Dr. Pressman on Health* on WEVD (1050 AM-NY). He is currently the director of Gramercy Health Associates in New York City.

Herbert D. Goodman, M.D., Ph.D., F.A.D.E.P., is a noted medical practitioner of both traditional and alternative medicine. His specialties include emergency medicine, pain management, acupuncture, geriatrics, and hypnosis.

Dr. Goodman is a Fellow in the American Academy of Disability Evaluating Physicians, a diplomate in the American Academy of Pain Management, and was elected as an approved consultant for the American Society of Clinical Hypnosis. He is currently director of the Southwestern Center for Pain in Phoenix, Arizona.

TITLES IN *THE PHYSICIANS' GUIDES* SERIES

From Berkley Books

THE PHYSICIANS' GUIDES TO HEALING

TREATING DIGESTIVE CONDITIONS

*Alan Pressman, D.C., Ph.D., D.A.C.B.N., C.C.N.,
and Herbert D. Goodman, M.D., Ph.D.,
with Sheila Buff*

Developed by The Philip Lief Group, Inc.

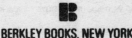

BERKLEY BOOKS, NEW YORK

This book is meant to educate and should not be used as an alternative to proper medical care. No treatments mentioned herein should be taken without qualified medical consultation and approval. The authors have exerted every effort to ensure that the information presented is accurate up to the time of publication. However, in light of ongoing research and the constant flow of information, it is possible that new findings may invalidate some of the data presented here.

TREATING DIGESTIVE CONDITIONS

A Berkley Book / published by arrangement with
The Philip Lief Group, Inc.

PRINTING HISTORY
Berkley edition / August 1997

The Putnam Berkley World Wide Web site address is
http://www.berkley.com

ISBN: 0-425-15940-X

BERKLEY®
Berkley Books are published by The Berkley Publishing Group,
200 Madison Avenue, New York, New York 10016.
BERKLEY and the "B" design are trademarks
belonging to Berkley Publishing Corporation.

PRINTED IN THE UNITED STATES OF AMERICA

10 9 8 7 6 5 4 3 2 1

Contents

Introduction

ARE YOU HEALTHY?

The answer to the above question may depend upon whom you ask. Allopathic medicine, also called conventional, traditional, or Western medicine, defines health as the absence of disease. In the allopathic tradition, chemical medications and surgical operations are the primary tools of healing. Much of the power to heal relies upon the progress of modern technology for its theories and practices. By contrast, holistic—also called alternative or natural medicine—is based on preventive care and focuses on not only bodily health but on psychological and spiritual health as well. To the holistic practitioner, good health is as much a reflection of our lifestyle and emotional stability as it is a product of avoiding disease and eating the proper foods. In the holistic vision of wellness, a balanced union of physical, spiritual, and emotional states produces vibrancy and longevity.

Clearly, allopathic and holistic practitioners approach health care from different vantage points. But there has been a revolution within the traditional medical establishment and a new era has begun—one that integrates alternative therapy and theories of overall wellness with allopathic medicine and rigorous practices of surgery and pharmaceuticals. Also known as complementary medicine, the fusion of the two schools of medicine has become the new frontier of health care. At last, patients can benefit from the collective wisdom of both ideologies of medical thought.

The *Physicians' Guides to Healing* series has been developed to give readers insight into the benefits of complementary medicine on a variety of health issues. The series consists of five authoritative health reference books, each of which provides accurate and up-to-date information on treatments from the perspectives of allopathic, alternative, and complementary medicine. The titles in the series—*Treating Asthma, Allergies, and Food Sensitivities; Treating Arthritis, Carpal Tunnel Syndrome, and Joint Conditions; Treating Hypertension and Other Cardiovascular Diseases; Treating Gynecological Conditions;* and *Treating Digestive Conditions*—will help the reader understand and compare both allopathic and alternative approaches to specific health problems, and make informed decisions about which combination of therapies is best suited to individual needs.

Dr. Herbert Goodman and Dr. Alan Pressman, coauthors of the series, lend their unsurpassed medical expertise to each volume. Both practitioners incorporate elements of natural medicine into their own traditional practices, approaching their patients' needs in a broad-minded and sensitive manner. Each book in the series reflects their confidence in complementary medicine and includes several case studies that closely examine the health problems and genuine concern of real people. These case histories demonstrate the potential healing power of complementary therapy when all else has failed, and they show how a candid and trusting relationship between doctor and patient is essential to effective and precise treatment.

Although the goals of both allopathic and alternative medicine are similar—health, immunity to diseases, and well-being—the approaches of holistic care focus more on preparing the body for a lifetime of total body health through healthy living, natural healing, and overall wellness rather than on curing specific illnesses as they arise. The various areas of alternative medicine include: mind/body control, as displayed in studies of art, dance, music therapy, biofeedback, yoga, and psychotherapy; manual healing therapies, such as acupressure, Alexander technique, chiropractic, massage, osteopathy, reflexology, and therapeutic touch; bioelectromagnetic therapy involving techniques such as blue light, artificial lighting, electrostimulation, and neuromagnetic stimulation; diet and nutrition, including vitamins, nutritional supplements, and practices like Gerson therapy; and herbal medicine, among other options. These are a few of the holistic remedies that you will become familiar with as you read the *Physicians' Guides to Healing*.

Of course, traditional treatments offer just as wide a range of possibilities and countless benefits. For instance, without the technology of modern surgical procedures and the mechanics of pacemakers, many people who suffer from irregular heartbeats would not be able to survive; likewise, without specialists' knowledge of orthopedic reconstruction operations, torn ligaments and deteriorated cartilage would prevent many injured people from walking. Cancerous tumors, including breast cancer, might claim the lives of thousands of cancer patients were it not for allopathic procedures such as mastectomies. Millions of cancer patients have extended their lives and improved their chances of survival with treatments such as surgery, radiation, and chemotherapy.

TRADITIONAL MEDICINE: A BRIEF HISTORY

Our knowledge of traditional medicine dates back as far as written history, although prescientific healing practices were based on magic, talismans, spells, incantations, and folk remedies ("old wives' tales"). Rudimentary surgery from the days before scientific medicine involved procedures such as trepanning, which entailed boring holes in the skull to relieve headaches, insanity, and epilepsy. As early as the third century B.C. doctors gained status as scientists, distinct from sorcerers and priests. Egyptian doctors are reported to have been trained for their profession by learning the arts of interrogation, inspection, and palpation (examination by touch). The drugs available to the Egyptians, though primitive, are still in use today, including figs, dates, and castor oil for laxative purposes; and tannic acid to soothe and treat burns. Early Mesopotamians also discovered a wealth of primitive pharmaceuticals in various forms, many of which were derived from mineral sources. The Mesopotamians are renowned for being the first society to develop accurate models of the liver, which they regarded as "the seat of the soul." This was the dawn of pharmacology, anatomy, and physiology.

The teachings of Hippocrates, the "father of medicine" who lived in Greece during the third century B.C., are the foundation of the modern medical values. His Hippocratic oath, which established a code of medical honor, is a vow of integrity that people in the health care industry take even today. Herophilus, an Egyptian from the same time period, is reported to have performed the first public dissection of a human cadaver. The founder of comparative anatomy was the Greek philosopher Aristotle, who also publicly performed dissections of many animals. According to etched records, early Egyptians performed castrations, removal of bladder stones, amputations, and various optical surgeries. Hindus in the second and third centuries A.D. performed the first known plastic surgery by grafting skin from the thigh and buttocks onto the nose. Chinese drugs in the same period included rhubarb, aconite, sulfur, animal organs, and—most importantly—opium, a powerful and effective pain reliever and anesthetic. The interest in the human body, the study of various types of life forms, and these early attempts at surgery and remedial drug use provided the foundations for the rest of medical evolution.

The Middle Ages in Europe were times of scientific advances as more empirical and physical knowledge accumulated among learned men. The Italians were the first people to officially separate science from religion in the ninth and tenth centuries, allowing progress to be propelled by research and analysis—not faith. In the thirteenth century, several countries including France and Italy saw the formation of the medieval guilds, which were social class rankings based upon profession. Barbers had always performed elementary surgery until the establishment of guilds. At that point, surgeons gained increased training, respect, and social status while barbers resigned themselves to haircutting and beard-shaving. In 1543, the publication of a treatise called *On the Structure of the Human Body* by the Belgian anatomist Andreas

Vesalius prompted a surge in medical research and the development of new physiological discoveries. In the same decade, colleagues and students of Vesalius made the first diagnoses of ear diseases and the identification of fallopian tubes, eye muscles, tear ducts, and they arrived at the notion of a circulatory system.

The most important milestone in seventeenth-century medicine was the discovery by English physician William Harvey, of the exact mechanism of blood circulation, a discovery that incited closer studies of the heart, lungs, and lymph systems as well. The introduction of quinine— a drug used to treat tuberculosis patients—was a major event in therapeutic progress during the seventeenth century. During this same period, French physician Ambroise Paré was nicknamed "the father of modern surgery" because he discovered that ligating arteries with a red-hot iron could be used to control bleeding and increase the patient's chances for survival. This discovery enabled doctors to perform surgery without worrying about time constraints or their patient's death from blood loss.

The notion of germs was taken quite seriously by nineteenth-century medical practitioners, and the use of carbolic acid (believed to kill germs) became a reliable way to reduce the likelihood of wound infections. Contributions to the understanding of shock management and antibiotic administration also greatly increased success rates in surgery. Other contributions from this century include X rays, discovered accidentally by Dr. Wilhelm Conrad Röntgen in Germany, and the use of ultraviolet radiation for treating many skin diseases, including psoriasis and tuberculosis of the skin. American scientists contributed significant research and understanding to operative gynecology: in 1809, Ephraim McDowell of

Kentucky performed the first successful removal of an ovarian tumor, marking the dawn of modern surgical procedure in the United States. Although medicine was rapidly achieving new and amazing goals, there were inevitable failures. For example, in the eighteenth century, John Brown promoted the theory that disease was caused by a lack of stimulation, and he therefore proposed stimulating his patients into health by bombarding them with "heroic" doses of poisonous drugs like mercuric chloride. Needless to say, not all of Dr. Brown's remedies resulted in restoring vigor and health to his patients.

The development of new ideas and technologies in the twentieth century has exponentially increased the magnitude of physical, chemical, surgical, and pharmacological knowledge. In addition to contributing to a general improvement in living conditions and a greater awareness of health issues, science has progressed into the realms of the previously inconceivable and impossible. For example, in the field of genetics, DNA replication is now possible; ultrasound technology makes viewing the fetus a normal prenatal procedure; and human life is readily created outside the woman's body by means of *in vitro* fertilization. And who would have believed that body parts could be reattached to the body, enabling dead tissue to come back to life? In 1962, the first successful limb replacement was performed: an arm, completely severed at the shoulder, was rejoined. Synthetic materials now allow surgeons to perform surgical replacements of hips, arms, teeth, and so on. Additionally, kidney and other organ transplants are now routinely successful.

Infectious diseases are largely under control now that most people have access to improved antibiotics, vaccines, and sanitation. The "wonder drugs" of the nineteenth and twentieth centuries have virtually wiped out most major diseases: sulfonamide antibiotics treat syphilis; streptomycin kills tuberculosis; sulfones treat leprosy; quinine treats malaria. Vaccines were developed for almost all of the most threatening epidemic diseases; for smallpox (1796), typhoid fever (1897), diphtheria (1923), tetanus (1930s) and for yellow fever, measles, mumps, and rubella. The discovery of penicillin in 1938 by Englishmen Howard Florey and Ernst Chain vastly reduced World War II fatalities and continues to effectively treat many types of infections. Genetic engineering, a concept that originated in the 1980s, led to the development of vaccines for herpes simplex, hepatitis B, influenza, and chicken pox. In general, scientists and physicians now have a vastly improved understanding of the human body's immune system and can therefore anticipate and eliminate most significant health hazards. Even with modern-day health horrors such as AIDS, the Ebola virus, and increased cancer incidence rates, we can have faith that science will eventually find more and better treatments for such diseases.

Cardiovascular disease, one of the most threatening contemporary medical conditions, has recently become less of an enigma thanks to imaging techniques like magnetic resonating imagery (MRI) developed in the 1970s. Cardiac catheterization, which enables measurements of pressure to be taken in the heart, helps doctors analyze potential heart conditions. Also, an array of drugs—including chemicals that have been developed to block certain functions of the sympathetic nervous system—is now available to treat angina, heart arrhythmia, and hypertension. Bypass surgery (replacing arteries damaged or narrowed by cholesterol buildup) and the transplantation of temporary and permanent artificial hearts have greatly widened options for sufferers of cardiovascular conditions. Such inventions and discoveries, complemented with essential nutritional information on reducing cholesterol, sodium, and fat intake, make controlling cardiovascular risk factors easier.

The new horizons in modern medicine promise a wealth of possibilities. Some practices that are now in their incipient stages with great promise for the future include cryogenics (freezing blood in surgeries such as those for Parkinson's disease and for brain tumors), psychopharmacology (which has virtually replaced the barbaric practice of prefrontal lobotomy), microsurgery (used, for example, to operate on the inner ear), the use of plastics (silicon and Teflon) to replace defective body parts, and transplantation (of teeth, liver, hearts, endocrine glands).

Modern medicine has evolved considerably since the days of trepanning, bloodletting with leeches, and induced purgation with mercuric chloride. Allopathic practitioners have begun to incorporate holistic therapies into their treatment programs, and they have accepted many of the ideas that were once only acknowledged by alternative practitioners, some of which are described below. The result: a progressive, preventive approach to healing, and the widely accepted conviction that complementary medicine works wonders. In 1992 the federal government established the Office of Alternative Medicine as part of the National Institutes of Health (NIH)—conclusive proof that alternative medicine has indeed entered the mainstream.

ALTERNATIVE MEDICINE: A BRIEF HISTORY

Natural medicine has always existed in various manifestations. Even before the advent of technological innovations and chemical research, human beings have taken the steps necessary to restore good health by using any remedy that appeared to positively affect their ailments. Long before modern pain medicine, Native Americans chewed on willow bark to relieve pain and headaches. Nowadays people are more likely to reach for a couple of aspirin tablets, but the principle is the same: willow contains salicylic acid, the same ingredient used to produce aspirin. We all want to drink ginger ale when we're feeling sick, but do you know the reason why? The properties of the herbal ginger root are known to settle stomachaches. Even if carbonated ginger ale hasn't been around for centuries, ginger tonic certainly has. The principles of natural healing have inspired many noninvasive cures for pain and illness throughout history. Throughout history Eastern medicine has been particularly successful in finding natural cures and using the body's inherent ability to heal itself from within. Much of what we consider "alternative" is simply Eastern in origin.

One of the oldest recorded alternative treatments is acupuncture, which dates back to 2000 B.C. Chinese healers developed acupuncture in response to the theory that there are special points known as meridians on the body connected to the internal organs and that vital energy flows along the lines that connect the meridians. According to this theory, diseases are caused by interruptions in the energy flow; inserting and twirling acupuncture needles into certain meridian points can stimulate energy and restore the body's normal energy flow. Acupuncture is widely used today in most Chinese hospitals for relieving pain, but only about 10 percent of American practitioners have recognized its efficacy and use it to treat patients. It is used as an analgesic for a wide variety of problems and is commonly employed in the treatment of brain surgery, ulcers, hypertension, asthma, and various heart conditions. The modern, physiological explanation for why and how acupuncture works, according to American neurophysiologists, is based on the theory that endorphins and enkephalins (the body's natural painkillers) are released when the skin is pierced by needles.

In the late eighteenth century, in defiance of the common medical procedure resulting from theories such as Dr. Brown's, Samuel Hahneman devised a theory that "likes are cured by likes," meaning that the body's natural defenses could be implemented to cure any ailment with the help of natural, botanical stimulants. Hahneman's theory was the birth of homeopathy as we know it today. His idea of using the elements already available to us in nature (such as chamomile flowers or Kombucha mushrooms) and within our own bodies (such as our highly complex and effective immune system) gave birth to a set of practices that continues to generate innovative techniques for holistic healing today. Homeopathy was introduced to the United States in 1825, and the American Institute of Homeopathy was founded in 1844.

An important milestone in the development of holistic medicine was the emergence of naturopathy, which means "natural curing." In 1902 a German doctor named Benedict Lust brought his theory of naturopathy to America. He had been impressed by the benefits he had witnessed in Europe when people who visited water spas would return refreshed, relaxed, and invigorated. He recognized that nature's abundant natural resources—like water and sun—could be tapped and utilized as great healing agents. Water curing has always been an effective therapeutic treatment; just think of relaxing in a hot tub or taking a long hot shower to unwind after a stressful day of work. The term *hydrotherapy* was coined shortly after Hahneman imported the idea to America. In some European countries today, a visit to the health spa for a water cure is covered by health insurance. Dr. Lust is responsible for a wider acceptance of natural medicine during his time than in any other period in modern medicine, present day excluded. He also believed in preventive measures such as good diet, exercise, mud baths, chiropractic massage, and other natural treatments. These fundamental tenets, along with Samuel Hahneman's, are still the cornerstones of holistic medicine today.

The major advancement of health care technology, especially in areas of surgery and pharmacology in the 1930s, is responsible for some of the deep segregation between homeopathic and traditional medicine. Earlier this century, there was virtually no way for homeopaths to spread the good word about such practices as hydrotherapy, botanical herbal treatments, or the benefits of massage—especially in the face of impressive medical and chemical breakthroughs in allopathic medicine. Chemical and drug companies had—and continue to have—a major financial stake in the promotion of allopathic medications and treatments; as a result, natural remedies have been brushed aside in a storm of advertising and promotion on the part of those larger drug companies and the allopathic practitioners who have advocated them.

Even the earliest homeopaths recognized the importance of regulating one's lifestyle as a highly important, controllable aspect of good health. Whether you are suffering from a medical condition or simply trying to improve the quality of your health, chances are you can feel better almost immediately by reducing your stress level. Learning to relax takes some time and effort, but the results of stress reduction benefit your cardiovascular system and your general sense of wellness. While most people need to work hard to accomplish goals at work, learning to take personal time to unwind and reflect should also be a priority. One method of learning to relax is biofeedback, which has proven helpful to patients with headaches, sore muscles, asthma complications, and stress-related problems. Hypnosis can induce a deeper contact with one's emotional life, resulting in the exposure of buried fears and conflicts and relief from repressions buried deep within the psyche. Massage methods such as reflexology and Swedish massage work miracles for relaxing tight muscles and loosening stiff necks that have been caused by hunching over a keyboard or spending long hours behind a desk. You will read about these and many other relaxation techniques in the *Physicians' Guides to Healing*.

Once you have mastered the art of relaxation, you will find it easier to make some more positive lifestyle changes. For instance, there's no time like the present if you've been intending to quit smoking or get in shape. Take a long walk. Make time to play outdoors with your children. Choose fresh fruit for dessert instead of pie. Use the stairs instead of the elevator. Wake up a few minutes early each morning to do some simple stretching. Physical activity will do a world of good and will make it much easier to change other bad habits into good ones. The small decisions you are faced with every day can turn into a set of healthy choices. Some alternative practitioners advocate hypnosis to correct behavioral difficulties such as smoking, overeating, and insomnia. Living an active, happy lifestyle free of harmful habits is one of the integral components of good health and a sense of overall vigor and vitality.

Besides lifestyle, one major element of health maintenance centers on diet and nutrition: a great deal of metabolic balance and general health depends on what foods we choose to put into our bodies. Nutrition was an inexact science until quite recently in this century. Nobody, including physicians and researchers, knew for certain what our bodies needed to subsist and flourish. The discovery of the existence of vitamins in the late nineteenth century prompted the theory that our bodies need three main types of nutrients to survive: food that builds and repairs tissue, food that can be burned for energy (calories), and food that regulates essential bodily functions.

For obvious reasons, both allopathic and alternative practitioners stress the importance of good diet. Feeding our bodies the wrong foods can promote cardiovascular disease, digestive stress, and general malaise. The government has developed a set of guidelines for proper nourishment and categorized them according to four major food groups: meat, vegetables, fruit, and dairy. Until the 1980s, a "balanced diet" consisted of equal amounts of each of these food groups, with an almost equal emphasis on meats and dairy products. While traditional medicine was inadvertently preaching this high-cholesterol, high-fat diet to the American public, holistic practitioners were advocating and enjoying the well-kept secret of vegetarianism and macrobiotics. To holistics, a balanced diet is one in which vegetables and grains prevail.

Nowadays the government guidelines for nutritional health have shifted away from the "four food group" grid in favor of a "food pyramid" in which the largest proportion of daily sustenance should be eaten from the grains category. The second largest category is fruits and vegetables. Then, smaller amounts of meat and poultry should be consumed, with the smallest daily servings in dairy and fats, oils, and sweets. There are more vegetarians—people who eat no red meat—and vegans—vegetarians who eat no animal products whatsoever, including eggs, cheese, and seafood—now than ever before; many people have discovered the benefits of eating low-fat and high-energy foods such as pasta, whole grains, and green leafy vegetables.

Another popular alternative approach to healing is chiropractic care, which is concerned with the relationship of the spinal column and the musculoskeletal structures of the body to the nervous system. The word "chiropractic" was derived from the Greek terms *cheir* (hand) and *praktikos* (practical). The main goal of chiropractic care is to help the body do its job. By correcting vertebral alignment, chiropractors minimize or eliminate interference to the normal flow of nerve energy throughout the body. This allows the body to repair its own systems and maintain good health without the use of drugs, surgery, or otherwise invasive medical procedures.

Chiropractic was conceived in an office building in Davenport, Iowa, in 1895. Its founder, Daniel David Palmer, noticed a bump on the neck of a janitor who, seventeen years earlier, had become suddenly and completely deaf when he had bent under a stairwell to reach for some cleaning supplies and had heard a prominent "snap." That noise was the last thing the man had heard for almost two decades. That is, until Daniel David Palmer pressed carefully on the janitor's bump and immediately restored normal hearing to the deaf man. With one firm jolt, chiropractic treatment had been born.

Chiropractic health care is now performed by licensed practitioners in all fifty states. Common conditions treated by chiropractic include headaches, neck pain, bronchial asthma, stress, nervous disorders, gastrointestinal disorders, respiratory conditions, strains, arthritis, and migraine headaches. A chiropractic adjustment is a rapid, precise force (referred to as dynamic thrust) to a specific point on the vertebra. When applied properly, it removes nerve interference and induces the body to respond with an appropriate healing reaction. A chiropractic manipulation is a nonspecific procedure that resets bones, increases range of movement, and realigns joint structure. Some chiropractors also offer such services as acupressure, nutrition counseling, herbal care and homeopathic treatments.

Members of the health care community have come to recognize that there is a place for alternative approaches such as chiropractic care, the alteration of nutritional choices, and reevaluation of lifestyles in our health-conscious society. Such alternative treatments as relaxation therapy, biofeedback, massage, nutritional and vitamin supplements, low-stress lifestyles, and hydrotherapy are now being prescribed by allopathic practitioners not only as preventive strategies, but as treatments for health disorders and conditions that already exist. For the active, overworked people of the 1990s, the wealth of new options available to patients and practitioners—thanks to the wider acceptance of homeopathy—have been embraced as welcome additions to the old, traditional set of choices. Consult your volumes in the *Physicians' Guides to Healing* series for a comprehensive introduction to the world of complementary medicine and for reliable, accurate answers to all your health-related questions.

THE PHYSICIANS' GUIDES TO HEALING

While homeopathy has been dismissed as "fringe" in the past and traditional medicine has prevailed, the past two decades have witnessed a movement back toward more natural and less invasive medical procedures. The benefits of both types of medicine are invaluable to complementary medical practitioners who treat patients with every disorder—from strokes and hypertension to hernias and ulcers; from hemorrhoids and rheumatoid arthritis to sprained joints; from urinary tract infections to menopausal discomfort, myocardial infarction, and seasonal hay fever. Who decides if you should use traditional treatments or alternative therapies? Is it necessary to choose between the two contrasting approaches, or can you safely combine them? How do you let your physician know your preferences? Is it possible for you to work as a team with your physician to determine how your symptoms should be treated, how your pain should be managed, and how long-term health may be maintained? The answers to all these questions, and many more, are readily available in each volume of the *Physicians' Guides to Healing* series.

CHAPTER 1

Introduction
to Digestive Conditions

Digestive problems of all sorts are extremely common. Many are minor and short-term, even though they may be unpleasant while they last. Fortunately, many digestive ailments can also be treated easily through diet and self-help steps. In fact, many treatments that would be considered alternative for other problems are standard medical practice for digestive problems. Even when they must prescribe medication to help a digestive problem such as gallstones, for example, physicians will also recommend dietary changes to help treat the problem and prevent future attacks. Another good example of a traditional dietary treatment is the role of dietary fiber in maintaining good digestive health. Long recognized as crucial by alternative practitioners, today most traditional practitioners recommend a high-fiber diet to their patients as well.

In this volume, diet and self-help steps are presented in the discussion of traditional treatments for digestive problems. Alternative treatments here are truly complementary. For example, one part of the dietary treatment for an ailment might be adding fiber. In the discussion of alternative treatments, we might suggest juices or herbal supplements as natural ways to increase your fiber intake. Similarly, we often recommend drinking six to eight eight-ounce glasses of pure water or other liquids, such as juices and herbal teas, as a traditional treatment—a suggestion that in other books might be given as an alternative hydrotherapy treatment for ailments not related to the digestive system.

Although many people think of chiropractic treatment only for the treatment of muscular and skeletal aches and pains, chiropractic treatment can be very helpful for some digestive ailments. As shown by numerous recent studies, there is a neural connection between the spinal cord and the digestive organs. Vertebral subluxations or misalignments can lower and diminish the activity of the stomach and intestines. In other words, these spinal lesions compromise the intestinal walls and play a major role in gastrointestinal dysfunction. Because of the spinal connection, various chiropractic reflex techniques are valuable adjuncts in treating gastrointestinal disorders. Chiropractic adjustments should concentrate on the misaligned vertebrae and also the principal vertebrae that may directly affect the intestinal organs: the third cervical, sixth and seventh dorsal, and fourth lumbar.

In the second chapter of this book, we discuss heartburn and indigestion, extremely common digestive problems that afflict almost everyone now and then. Chronic heartburn, also called gastroesophageal reflux disease (GERD) is a surprisingly common and often undiagnosed problem. Fortunately, health care providers today are much more aware of GERD and now have much better ways to treat it. In the past few years, effective drugs called H_2 blockers have been developed to treat heartburn and GERD. These drugs, including Zantac, Pepcid, and Axid, are so safe and so valuable that they have been approved for over-the-counter sales. In addition to such drugs, however, dietary measures, herbal remedies, and other alternative treatments are often very helpful for heartburn and indigestion.

Nausea and vomiting, traced to a variety of causes, are discussed in chapter 3. Dietary steps, herbal remedies, acupressure, and other alternative treatments are particularly helpful for nausea. Morning sickness, for example, is often relieved quite a bit by simple dietary steps and mild herbal teas. One of the most valuable uses of acupressure is in the treatment of motion sickness. Acupressure wristbands that press constantly on points in the wrist can often relieve even severe motion sickness.

In the past few years significant new discoveries have made peptic ulcer disease, the subject of chapter 4, far easier to diagnose and treat. In this chapter we discuss the bacterium that has been shown to be the cause of most ulcers and the new treatment methods that eradicate most ulcers quickly and easily. We also discuss dietary measures and alternative treatments that help relieve ulcer discomfort and aid in healing.

We discuss food allergies and sensitivities extensively in chapter 5. We believe that undiagnosed food sensitivities may be the root cause of many other digestive problems and may even be a hidden cause of other health problems such as arthritis. For this reason, we include an extensive discussion of how food intolerances are diagnosed. We also discuss leaky gut syndrome, a condition that allows undigested food particles to enter the bloodstream, which can trigger allergic responses with a variety of unpleasant symptoms.

Leaky gut syndrome is covered more thoroughly in chapter 6, where we discuss common problems of the small intestine. Although leaky gut syndrome can be the underlying cause of a large number of common digestive ailments, many traditional health care providers don't consider it when diagnosing their patients. Alternative practitioners have much to offer here. In this chapter we also discuss dysbiosis, or bacterial overgrowth of the small intestine. Dysbiosis too may be an underlying cause of other problems, including leaky gut syndrome. Here, too, traditional health care providers have been slow to accept how widespread the problem is. Alternative methods can often diagnose the problem and cure it gently. Pancreatic insufficiency is another digestive problem that is perhaps more common than traditional practitioners realize. Here, too, alternative treatments often help relieve many of the digestive symptoms.

In chapter 7 we discuss the painful problem of gallstones. Diet is particularly important for treating gallbladder attacks and preventing recurrences. Many traditional herbal remedies and other alternative treatments are also quite helpful. For serious cases, however, medication or even surgery to remove the gallbladder must be considered. Modern surgery for gallbladder removal uses fiber optics and miniaturized instruments. What was once a major surgical operation with a long and painful recovery period is now much easier on the patient.

Chapter 8 is a thorough discussion of the three common bowel problems: gas, diarrhea, and constipation. Because these are ailments that almost everyone has now and then, large amounts of drugstore shelf space are devoted to over-the-counter remedies. But diet and self-help steps, along with alternative treatments, are simpler, gentler, more effective, and less expensive. In this chapter we also discuss the often overlooked problem of intestinal parasites.

More serious problems of the large intestine are discussed in chapter 9. We begin with a long discussion of the toxic bowel and the vital role of dietary fiber in digestive health. The concept of the toxic bowel is one that traditional health care providers are accepting more and more, although alternative practitioners are still more likely to diagnose the problem quickly and accurately. Curing a toxic bowel problem often clears up other persistent digestive problems and may also help other chronic health problems. Irritable bowel syndrome and inflammatory bowel diseases such as ulcerative colitis and Crohn's disease are also discussed in this chapter. In many cases, irritable bowel syndrome responds particularly well to diet, dietary fiber, and alternative treatments. Inflammatory bowel diseases are more difficult to treat and often require powerful medications to control flare-ups. Once the flare-ups are under control, however, relapses can often be prevented through careful attention to diet and some alternative treatments.

We end the book with a discussion of hemorrhoids, an extremely common problem. Here again dietary fiber is vital for preventing and treating the ailment. Self-help steps, hydrotherapy treatments such as sitz baths, and alternative methods are often very helpful for dealing with the symptoms.

ABOUT HOMEOPATHIC REMEDIES

Homeopathy is based on the principle, first expounded by the German physician Samuel Hahnemann in the late 1700s, that like cures like. In other words, Hahnemann believed that a drug that causes symptoms similar to a particular disease could also cure that disease, but only if given in very tiny doses. The homeopathic dose is said to stimulate the patient's vital force and help him or her fight off the illness. In the nineteenth century, others expanded on Hahnemann's ideas and added more remedies.

In homeopathic theory, the more dilute a remedy is, paradoxically, the more potent it is. In general, low potency remedies are used for acute problems, while high potency remedies are used for chronic conditions. The potency of a homeopathic remedy is indicated by a numeral and the letter x (for liquids) or c (for solids) following the remedy name. The number indicates the number of times the basic plant or mineral extract in the remedy has been diluted. The basic extract is diluted one part extract to nine parts water and then succussed (shaken vigorously and rhythmically) to give a 1x dilution, meaning one part in ten. This mixture is then diluted and succussed again to make a 2x dilution, or one part in one hundred. The mixture is then usually diluted and succussed several more times to make the most common homeopathic dose, 6x (6c if the mixture is combined with lactose to make a pill). A 6x dose of a homeopathic remedy contains one part of the basic extract to one million parts water.

Homeopathic remedies are readily available in health food stores and well-stocked pharmacies. The labels on the remedies can be a little strange and confusing. The name of the remedy is generally given in abbreviated form according to the standard homeopathic system. *Carbo veg.*, for example, is the abbreviated form of carbo vegetabilis, the Latin term used by homeopaths for charcoal.

Tissue salts, also sometimes called Schüssler tissue salts, cell salts, or biochemic salts, are homeopathic preparations of one or more of a dozen minerals found in the human body. Some tissue salts are available as single salts such as mag. phos. (magnesium phosphate). Many people prefer to purchase premixed combinations. Combination Q, for example, contains ferrum phos. (iron phosphate), kali mur. (potassium chloride), kali sulf. (potassium sulfate), and natrum mur. (sodium chloride)—a combination said to help sinus problems, colds, and flu.

Because they are so dilute, homeopathic remedies can be given frequently. Most homeopaths suggest up to seven consecutive doses, spaced anywhere from ten to thirty minutes apart. After the maximum number of doses, wait three to four hours before beginning again. Homeopathic remedies can generally be used safely in conjunction with whatever medications or other steps a traditional physician recommends. They should not, however, be used instead of standard drug treatment for a diagnosed medical problem.

Use homeopathic remedies only to treat minor ailments. Delays in seeking needed medical treatment can lead to serious complications. If you take a homeopathic remedy and do not get better within a couple of days, or if you get worse, see your doctor. If the problem recurs, see your doctor. If you suddenly get much worse, see your doctor at once.

CHAPTER 2

Heartburn and Indigestion

Almost all of us occasionally get heartburn or indigestion from something we've eaten or drunk. In most cases, the problem causes some minor discomfort and goes away fairly soon on its own, or with a little help from some easy self-treatment steps. For some 32 million Americans, however, heartburn is a chronic problem that causes severe discomfort.

Because heartburn and indigestion are such common problems, they have many effective traditional and alternative treatments. For occasional heartburn and indigestion, select the treatment that works best for you. If you have persistent heartburn or indigestion that doesn't respond to the treatments discussed below, or if the problem is getting worse, see your health care provider.

HEARTBURN

Heartburn—a painful burning sensation in your upper abdomen or lower chest, often accompanied by a sour taste in the back of your throat—is one of the most common digestive problems. Despite its name, heartburn doesn't have anything to do with your heart. It's actually your esophagus that's the source of the discomfort.

Your esophagus is a ten-inch tube that connects your mouth to your stomach. When you eat, food travels down your esophagus and passes through a ringlike opening, called the lower esophageal sphincter (LES), to enter your stomach. The lower esophageal sphincter is basically a one-way valve that opens to let in the food and then closes tightly shut again to keep the powerful hydrochloric acid of your digestive juices safely inside the stomach. Sometimes, however, the LES doesn't close completely or doesn't stay closed. Stomach acid can then back up (reflux) into your esophagus. Not surprisingly, the acid causes a very uncomfortable burning sensation when it comes in contact with the unprotected lining of your esophagus. The burning sensation also gives heartburn another name, acid stomach.

Almost everyone experiences mild heartburn every now and then, usually from eating too much or eating too quickly. The discomfort can be severe, but it usually passes fairly quickly and doesn't return—at least until the next time you overeat or grab a meal on the run. Some people get heartburn from eating particular foods that relax the sphincter muscles and make reflux more likely, or from eating foods that stimulate the stomach to make more acid, which can also lead to reflux. Alcoholic beverages cause heartburn for some people. Some prescription drugs, especially beta blockers and calcium channel blockers, can cause heartburn as a side effect. Even if you think your medicine is causing your heartburn, don't stop taking it. Talk to your doctor instead—you may be able to switch to a different drug. Pregnant women often suffer from heartburn, perhaps because pregnancy makes the LES close less tightly and perhaps because the growing fetus puts pressure on the abdomen.

At one time physicians believed that hiatus hernia, a condition in which part of the stomach pushes up through the diaphragm and into the chest, was the main cause of heartburn. Hiatus hernias are very common, however, and most people who have them don't get heartburn any more than anyone else—and most people who frequently get heartburn don't have hiatus hernias.

Some people get frequent heartburn even when they're careful about what and how they eat and drink. For unknown reasons, they simply have weak lower esophageal sphincters and get heartburn more often than others.

Of the 32 million Americans who suffer from chronic heartburn, less than half have ever mentioned their problem to a health care provider. If you often get severe heartburn, don't assume that it's caused by something you ate or that you just have to live with it. You may have a more severe digestive problem such as a duodenal ulcer or gastroesophageal reflux disease (GERD). Because GERD is usually very uncomfortable, and because it can lead to esophageal ulcers, a precancerous condition called Barrett's esophagus, esophageal scarring, hoarseness, and possibly asthma, see your doctor if your severe heartburn is persistent or doesn't respond to the nondrug treatments we discuss below. If you think your heartburn is caused by an ulcer, see the discussion later in this book.

The pain of heartburn is sometimes so severe that it is mistaken for a heart attack. Even worse, sometimes heart attack pain is dismissed as just heartburn. If you have heartburn pain so severe that it makes you break out into a sweat, or if the pain extends from your chest into your neck or left shoulder or arm, or if the pain is accompanied by a crushing or viselike sensation in the chest, you might be having a heart attack. Let a trained professional decide what's causing the pain—get emergency medical help at once.

Traditional Treatments

Occasional heartburn responds extremely well to traditional treatments, including dietary measures, self-help steps, and over-the-counter antacids. More serious heartburn and GERD also respond well to these treatments, but they may also need additional treatment with prescription medications.

Diet   The goal of treating heartburn through diet is to avoid foods that relax the LES, irritate the esophagus, and increase the production of stomach acid. Foods that relax the LES and make reflux more likely will vary from person to person, but common culprits include chocolate, fatty or fried foods, dairy foods, cream sauces, nuts, and peppermint. Avoid alcohol and beverages containing caffeine. The spice in spicy foods is rarely the real cause of heartburn. If you get heartburn after eating pepperoni pizza, for example, it is probably because of the fat in the pepperoni, not the hot pepper. However, if your esophagus is already irritated from heartburn, spicy or acidic foods such as hot peppers, tomato sauce, or orange juice could irritate it further. Any beverage containing caffeine stimulates the production of stomach acid—and so does decaffeinated coffee. Alcoholic or carbonated beverages also rev up stomach acid.

If you often get heartburn after eating a specific food, even if it's not one of the foods discussed above, that food is a trigger for you. To avoid heartburn, avoid the food.

Self-help steps Heartburn can be avoided, at least some of the time, with some simple self-help steps. If you smoke, stop. If alcoholic beverages give you heartburn, cut back on your drinking. Many of our patients find that eating smaller, more frequent meals helps their heartburn quite a bit. So does eating more slowly and chewing your food thoroughly.

If you are overweight, especially if you carry the weight around your waist, losing some pounds will probably reduce your incidence of heartburn. The extra weight puts pressure on your abdomen and the lower esophageal sphincter. For the same reason, avoid wearing tight clothes that press on the abdomen.

Moderate exercise after eating, such as walking a mile or two at a normal pace, may aid digestion and prevent heartburn, but avoid vigorous exercise just after a meal.

Don't bend over or lie down immediately after eating—these positions make it much easier for acid to flow upward. Since most people produce a lot of stomach acid at night while they sleep, try to avoid eating for at least three hours before bedtime. To help prevent reflux while you sleep, try elevating the head of your bed by at least six inches (many people use bricks or blocks). This raises your torso, and hence your LES, above your stomach. You'll have less reflux because the stomach acid has to flow uphill. One of our patients hadn't had a full night's sleep in several years—heartburn would invariably wake him three hours after he went to sleep. Elevating the head of his bed worked a near miracle. If raising the bed is inconvenient (your bed partner may object), you can purchase a wedge-shaped pillow that has the same effect. Just sleeping with a lot of pillows won't really help—you need to elevate not just your head but your whole torso to prevent reflux.

Antacids As their name suggests, antacids neutralize the powerful acid in your stomach and relieve the burning sensation it causes when it backs up into your esophagus. Interestingly, your own saliva contains a natural antacid. If you feel heartburn coming on, try sucking on a hard candy (not a mint, which will relax the esophageal sphincter) or chewing gum. This will stimulate you to produce extra saliva that may put out the fire.

If stronger measures are needed, try one of the many nonprescription antacids available as chewable tablets or as liquids. Both forms generally work quickly and effectively, although the liquids usually work a little faster.

You should be aware, however, that antacids can interfere with the actions of some drugs. If you are taking any prescription medications (particularly antibiotics, anticoagulants, or medications for angina or high blood pressure) or have kidney disease, talk to your doctor before taking an antacid. If you have heartburn because you are pregnant, talk to your doctor about antacids.

Antacids contain acid-neutralizing substances such as sodium bicarbonate, calcium carbonate, magnesium hydroxide, or aluminum hydroxide, singly or in combination. Antacids should be used in conjunction with the self-help and dietary measures discussed above, not instead of them.

Drinking half a teaspoon of sodium bicarbonate (the chemical name for baking soda) stirred into half a glass of water is a traditional and effective home remedy for occasional heartburn. Sodium bicarbonate is the active ingredient in fizzy heartburn remedies such as Alka-Seltzer, Bromo-Seltzer, and Brioschi. Alka-Seltzer contains aspirin, however, which can irritate your stomach. In general, antacids containing sodium bicarbonate should be used only occasionally, since they can disrupt your body's acid balance and may lead to urinary tract infections. If you should restrict the amount of sodium in your diet, avoid these antacids.

Magnesium hydroxide, the active ingredient in antacids such as Maalox, Mylanta, milk of magnesia, Di-Gel, Riopan, and many other products, is a very effective heartburn reliever. By itself, magnesium hydroxide causes diarrhea, so almost all magnesium antacid formulations also contain aluminum hydroxide to counterbalance the laxative effect. Even so, large or frequent doses of a magnesium-aluminum antacid can give you diarrhea. Large doses can also be dangerous if you have kidney disease. We usually recommend magnesium-based antacids to our patients for the short-term treatment of occasional mild to moderately severe heartburn—they're quick, effective, and safe.

Aluminum-based antacids such as Rolaids or Amphojel are effective heartburn relievers, but they are slower and less potent than aluminum-magnesium compounds. Aluminum hydroxide can be constipating, so these products usually contain some magnesium as a counterbalance. Despite this, frequent use of aluminum-based antacids can lead to constipation. There is, by the way, no evidence that links the aluminum in antacids to the development of Alzheimer's disease later in life.

Antacids vary in their ability to neutralize acid. Generally speaking, magnesium-aluminum liquid antacids, especially those that have the numeral or word "two" or the word "plus" in their names, are the most potent and will be most effective for relieving heartburn. We usually recommend Maalox Plus, Mylanta II, or their generic equivalents, to our patients.

How much of an antacid should you take, and when should you take it? There are no hard and fast rules. Most of our patients find that taking two antacid tablets or one or two tablespoons of liquid antacid as soon as they feel the first symptoms helps stop heartburn quickly. If you don't get relief within ten minutes or so, take another dose or even a third—it can take a lot of antacid to neutralize a stomach full of hydrochloric acid. If heartburn wakes you in the night, take a dose of antacid before you go to sleep.

If you find yourself taking frequent large doses of antacids, if the antacids don't help your heartburn for long, if you have persistent heartburn for more than two weeks, if you have trouble swallowing or have persistent abdominal pain, if you vomit blood, or if your stools are bloody or black, you may have a more serious problem. See your doctor at once.

Drugs In recent years the treatment of severe heartburn, GERD, and ulcers has been vastly improved by the development of two new types of drugs. H_2 blockers, drugs that sharply reduce the stomach's acid production by blocking the effects of histamine, were introduced in the late 1970s. Tagamet, the first of these drugs, became the most widely prescribed drug in the world within a year. Other H_2 blockers such as Zantac, Pepcid, and Axid quickly came on the market; Zantac has now been prescribed over 200 million times worldwide. Sir James Black, the discoverer of H_2 blockers, received the Nobel prize in 1988.

All the H_2 blockers are generally very safe and only very rarely have any side effects. In fact, these drugs are so effective and so safe that they are now available in nonprescription form. The usual dose is one or two tablets taken with water as soon as symptoms begin, up to twice daily. However, if nonprescription H_2 blockers don't help your heartburn for long, if you have persistent heartburn for more than two weeks, if you have trouble swallowing or have persistent abdominal pain, if you vomit blood, or if your stools are bloody or black, you may have a more serious problem. See your doctor at once.

Soon after H_2 blockers were discovered, researchers in Sweden discovered a compound that went one step beyond blocking stomach acid production—they found a drug, called omeprazole, that turns off acid production altogether. It wasn't until 1989, however, that the drug, marketed under the brand name Prilosec, became available. Prilosec has revolutionized the treatment of severe heartburn and gastroesophageal reflux disease. It is very safe, very effective, and easy to take—just one pill every morning before breakfast.

Surgery In very severe cases of intractable heartburn that do not respond to medication, surgery to tighten the lower esophageal sphincter may be recommended. Recent improvements in microsurgery techniques make this operation less serious than it once was, but the surgery does not always succeed and there is a fairly large risk of undesirable side effects. This surgery is usually recommended only if all else, including Prilosec, has failed.

Severe hiatus hernias causing intractable symptoms can also be surgically repaired. Again, this is a serious operation that is recommended only as a last resort.

Alternative Treatments

Acupressure/acupuncture   The traditional acupressure point for heartburn is conception vessel (CV) 12, which is located on your abdomen about halfway between your belly button and your breastbone. Apply gentle pressure for two minutes, preferably on an empty stomach. A trained acupuncturist will treat heartburn and digestive problems by releasing the energy of the spleen and other energy points related to the digestive system.

In traditional shiatzu (Japanese acupressure), heartburn may be relieved by massaging the legs. Sit on the floor with your knees drawn up and your feet flat on the floor. Place your left thumb in the bend of your right knee; your left fingers will be resting on your shin. The shiatzu point you want to massage is on the outside of your right calf about where your left middle finger is pointing. Massage the point gently for ten to twenty seconds, then repeat twice more. Repeat three times on your left leg with your right hand.

Reflexology   Gently massaging the stomach reflexes of the hands and feet can help relieve heartburn symptoms. If you frequently get heartburn, regular massage in these areas might help reduce the frequency and severity of your symptoms. The stomach reflexes of each hand are found on the palm, in the area below the pads of the index and middle fingers. On each foot, the stomach reflexes are on the sole, in the area just below the large pad of the big toe. Some reflexologists believe that massaging the diaphragm and solar plexus reflex points of the hands and feet also helps heartburn. These points overlap, on both hands, in the palm, just below the pad of the middle finger. They also overlap on the sole just below the ball of the foot.

Chiropractic treatments   Chiropractic adjustment by a trained chiropractor is often very helpful for cases of persistent heartburn, especially if a hiatus hernia is the cause.

Herbal therapy   A number of herbal teas are traditionally recommended for heartburn. Strong chamomile, meadowsweet, or lemon balm tea helps many people. Teas made from caraway, anise, or fennel seeds are also safe and effective for relieving heartburn; they all have a characteristic "licorice" flavor. Some people swear by tea made from dill seeds. To try these remedies, make the tea by crushing a teaspoonful of the seeds and steeping it in one cup of boiling water for fifteen minutes. Strain before drinking; sip the teas slowly for maximum relief.

In traditional Chinese herbal medicine, a cup of ginger tea is often recommended for quick relief of heartburn. Steep one teaspoon of finely chopped fresh ginger in one cup of boiling water for ten minutes. Strain before drinking; sip the tea slowly for maximum relief.

Traditional Ayurvedic medicine recommends a tea made from ground bay leaf for heartburn relief. Steep half a teaspoon of the ground bay leaf in one cup of boiling water for ten minutes. Strain before drinking; sip the tea slowly for maximum relief.

Juice therapy   Banana juice—or just eating a banana— is often very helpful for relieving heartburn. Since bananas don't juice very well, combine one peeled banana with one cup of pear or apple juice in the juicer or blender. Drinking the mixture may relieve your heartburn almost immediately.

Just as tea made from fennel seeds can help heartburn, so too can juice made from the fennel stem. The feathery cap of leaves makes fennel look a bit like dill. Fennel is an excellent source of vitamin A, potassium, and dietary fiber. To make fennel juice, remove the leaves and rinse the stems thoroughly. Juice the stems. If you find the anise flavor too strong, add some carrot juice to the mixture. If you frequently get heartburn after eating, try slowly sipping a quarter cup of fresh fennel juice shortly before eating. If you already have heartburn, slowly sip a quarter cup of the juice. If the heartburn persists, try another quarter cup.

Hydrotherapy   One of the simplest and most effective remedies for heartburn is to slowly sip a glass of cool water. The water washes the stomach acid out of your esophagus. Another useful remedy is activated charcoal, easily available at health food stores and well-stocked pharmacies. Mix two tablespoons of activated charcoal with one ounce of cool water in a twelve-ounce glass. When the mixture is well blended, slowly stir in enough water to fill the glass. Sip the mixture through a straw. Alternatively, swallow two activated charcoal tablets with a glass of water. Use activated charcoal only occasionally—frequent use can lead to impaired digestion.

Many people who get frequent heartburn claim that they can prevent it by drinking a glass of water mixed with one tablespoon of lemon juice or cider vinegar about an hour before meals. Another remedy that seems to help some people is raw potato juice, diluted half and half with water.

Homeopathic remedies   Several homeopathic remedies are suggested for heartburn. For simple heartburn or
"acid stomach," the tissue salt (mineral) nat. phos. 6x is
usually recommended. Take it every five to ten minutes
if the heartburn is severe; otherwise, take it every thirty
minutes until the symptoms go away. If the heartburn is
accompanied by bloating or gas, try carbo veg. 30c every
ten to fifteen minutes; repeat up to seven times. If you
have heartburn and severe gas, try argentum nit. 6c every
three to four hours. For heartburn accompanied by nausea, try pulsatilla 6c every ten to fifteen minutes; repeat
up to seven times. Late-night heartburn occurring several hours after eating may be relieved by arsen. alb. 6c
every three to four hours. For indigestion from overeating, and especially from too much rich, fatty food, try
pulsatilla 6c every ten to fifteen minutes until the discomfort passes; take no more than seven doses in total.
Alternatively, try carbo veg. 30c every ten to fifteen minutes until the discomfort passes; take no more than seven
doses in total. If excessive gas or bloating accompanies
the indigestion, try carbo veg. 6c every half hour; take no
more than ten doses in total. The tissue salt kali mur. 6x
every three to four hours may help. If your indigestion is
accompanied by nausea, try ant. crud. 6c every three to
four hours.

Relaxation techniques   Gulping down of food is a
common cause of heartburn. Try to have your meals in a
pleasant, relaxed environment. Eat slowly and chew each
mouthful thoroughly. Yoga exercises that help tone the
digestive system and abdominal area may help.

Combined Treatments

Antacids and acupressure/acupuncture   If you often suffer from severe heartburn, antacids or other remedies are needed to relieve the immediate discomfort. Acupuncture and acupressure can be very helpful for reducing the frequency and severity of the attacks.

Antacids and herbal therapy   Because long-term use of antacids can lead to diarrhea or constipation, we often suggest trying an herbal tea for mild heartburn and moving on to an antacid only if the tea gives no relief.

Antacids and relaxation   Many patients suffer from heartburn because their high-stress lives never allow them to just relax and enjoy their meals. Instead, they gulp their food, jolt themselves awake with caffeine, and then spend nights in misery from heartburn. Antacids can relieve heartburn symptoms, but only learning to relax and eat slowly will help prevent heartburn in these cases.

INDIGESTION

Indigestion (sometimes called dyspepsia) is a catchall term for unpleasant sensations of fullness, pressure, churning, bloating, cramping, gassiness, "repeating," and the like in the stomach. Indigestion can have many causes, but it is almost always brought on by eating too quickly or too much, from stress, or from eating foods that "disagree" with you. Sometimes indigestion is caused by a prescription medication. If you think that is the case, discuss your medication with your doctor. And if you have indigestion that doesn't go away within a few days, call your doctor.

Indigestion that makes you feel full or bloated may be caused by too little hydrochloric acid in the stomach (hypochlorhydria). The presence of hydrochloric acid stimulates your stomach to produce pepsin, the major digestive juice, and it also stimulates the pyloric valve leading to the small intestine to open. If you don't produce enough hydrochloric acid, you may not produce enough pepsin, which in turn could lead to frequent indigestion. Other symptoms of hypochlorhydria include bad breath, constipation, and undigested food in the stools. Since hydrochloric acid kills bacteria and other pathogens, having a low acid level could make you more vulnerable to digestive problems such as ulcers, gastritis, gastroenteritis, and food poisoning.

Hypochlorhydria symptoms can sometimes be similar to those of heartburn, even though their causes are exactly opposite, so you need to know which condition is causing the problem. If antacids quickly relieve your discomfort, heartburn is almost certainly the culprit. If swallowing one or two tablespoons of cider vinegar or lemon juice relieves your discomfort, hypochlorhydria may be the cause. For a more accurate diagnosis, speak to your health care provider about taking a gastro capsule test or having a Heidelberg gastrogram.

Most people gradually produce less hydrochloric acid as they age, and they suffer no ill effects from the change; people who take H_2 blockers or Prilosec for long periods also seem to suffer no side effects from producing little or no hydrochloric acid. It's possible that infection with the *Helicobacter pylori* bacteria, which causes gastritis and gastric ulcers, may also lead to lowered hydrochloric acid levels. (For more information about *H. pylori* infection, see chapter 4 on peptic ulcer disease.)

Another major source of indigestion is gas (otherwise known as burping, belching, or eructation). Stomach gas is almost always caused by swallowed air, not by gas-producing foods such as cabbage or beans—the gas they cause occurs lower down, in the large intestine.

Traditional Treatments

Diet   Trigger foods for indigestion are often the same as those for heartburn, as discussed above. Foods that are high in protein or fat make your stomach secrete more digestive juices, which in turn can cause indigestion. If you often feel indigestion symptoms after a protein-rich or fatty meal, try cutting back and eating more carbohydrates, vegetables, and fruits instead. Lactose intolerance (the inability to digest milk) can cause indigestion symptoms, especially gas and cramping. (See the section on lactose intolerance in chapter 5 for more information.) Alcohol, caffeine, and carbonated beverages can also cause indigestion.

Gas can be avoided by reducing the amount of air you swallow. Avoid carbonated beverages. Chewing gum and sucking candies can also cause you to swallow excess air. Avoid drinking a lot of liquids with meals. Eat slowly and chew your food thoroughly.

Some people simply find that certain foods "disagree" with them. One of our patients got indigestion from cucumbers (but not pickles) and green bell peppers (but not jalapeño peppers). She cured the problem by avoiding those foods. If you often get indigestion, try keeping a food diary that records what you ate at each meal and whether you got indigestion within a few hours of eating.

If you do have any trigger foods for indigestion, the food diary could help pinpoint them. On the other hand, if you have symptoms more severe than mild indigestion after eating a particular food, or if your symptoms occur more than a few hours after eating, you may have a food allergy or intolerance. (See chapter 5 on food allergies for more information.)

Angostura bitters or traditional aperitifs such as Campari taken shortly before eating help stimulate the flow of hydrochloric acid in the stomach.

Self-help steps   The same self-help steps that help heartburn also help indigestion. Moderate exercise such as a walk after meals often helps move gas up and out of the stomach and also stimulates the flow of hydrochloric acid. Smoking and drinking alcohol are both causes of indigestion. If you smoke, stop or at least avoid cigarettes just before eating. If alcoholic beverages give you indigestion, cut back.

Medication   If your indigestion is accompanied by heartburn, the antacids discussed above may help relieve your symptoms. Indigestion without heartburn is often helped by taking one to three tablespoons of pink bismuth (Pepto-Bismol) liquid. Indigestion from stomach gas can be relieved with an over-the-counter drug called simethicone, which helps break up gas bubbles. Some over-the-counter liquid antacids also contain simethicone. Look for products labeled "antacid/anti-gas." Low-acidity can be treated with supplements of hydrochloric acid in the form of glutamic acid hydrochloride (glutamic acid HCL) or betaine hydrochloride with pepsin. Start by taking one capsule in either form with each main meal, then increase the dosage gradually by one capsule to a maximum of three capsules per meal. Cut back if you feel a warm or burning sensation in the stomach, have stomach pain, or feel nauseous.

Alternative Treatments

Acupressure/acupuncture   The traditional acupressure point for indigestion is the same as for heartburn: conception vessel (CV) 12, which is located on your abdomen about halfway between your belly button and your breastbone. Apply gentle pressure for two minutes, preferably on an empty stomach.

In traditional shiatzu (Japanese acupressure), indigestion may be relieved by massaging the legs. Sit on the floor with your knees drawn up and your feet flat on the floor. Place your left thumb in the bend of your right knee; your left fingers will be resting on your shin. The shiatzu point you want to massage is on the outside of your right calf about where your left middle finger is pointing. Massage the point gently for ten to twenty seconds, then repeat twice more. Repeat three times on your left leg with your right hand.

A trained acupuncturist will treat frequent indigestion by releasing the energy of the spleen and other energy points related to the digestive system.

Reflexology   Gently massaging the stomach reflexes of the hands and feet can help relieve indigestion. If you frequently get indigestion, a regular massage in these areas might help reduce the frequency and severity of your symptoms. The stomach reflexes of each hand are found on the palm, in the area below the pads of the index and middle fingers. On each foot, the stomach reflexes are on the sole, in the area just below the large pad of the big toe.

Some reflexologists believe that massaging the diaphragm and solar plexus reflex points of the hands and feet also helps heartburn. These points overlap on each hand in the palm, just below the pad of the middle finger. They also overlap on the sole just below the ball of each foot.

Chiropractic treatments   Chiropractic adjustment by a trained chiropractor is often helpful for cases of persistent indigestion.

Herbal therapy   The herbal remedies for heartburn discussed above help indigestion and stomach gas as well. Other herbs that help relieve stomach or intestinal gas are called carminatives. If you have indigestion without heartburn, strong peppermint tea, for instance, may help. Herbs that help relieve stomach or intestinal gas are called carminatives. Peppermint and chamomile tea also often help stomach gas, but teas made from fennel or anise seem to work best. Other carminatives that may help include catnip (a type of mint) and cinnamon.

Traditional Chinese carminatives are teas made from ginseng or freshly grated ginger. Ginseng is usually taken as a tea made from the powdered root. To prepare ginseng tea, steep one to three teaspoons of ginseng in one cup of boiling water for ten minutes, stirring occasionally. Stir before drinking. To make ginger tea, steep one teaspoon of freshly grated or finely chopped fresh ginger in one cup of boiling water for ten minutes. Strain before drinking. Tea bags containing dried ginger can be bought at health food stores; these work almost as well as making your own tea from fresh ginger.

In India, a traditional remedy for indigestion is *chai ka masala*, or spiced tea. To make the spice mixture, you will need one-half teaspoon of cardamon seeds, one-quarter teaspoon of carom seeds (a tiny, fragrant seed available in ethnic groceries—but you can omit the carom if you can't find it), 6 cloves, one-half teaspoon of fennel seeds, 8 whole black peppercorns, one teaspoon of ground ginger, and one teaspoon of ground cinnamon. In a spice or coffee grinder, grind the cardamon seeds, carom seeds, cloves, fennel seeds, and peppercorns until fine. Add the ground ginger and cinnamon and mix well. Store in a tightly closed container in a cool, dark place; the mixture will stay fresh for six months. To make the actual *chai ka masala*, combine two and a half cups of pure water with one teaspoon of the spice mix in a saucepan. Bring to a boil over high heat. Reduce the heat, cover the saucepan, and simmer for five minutes. Add one to two teaspoons of loose black tea (or just a tea bag or two) and simmer for one minute longer. Strain into cups.

If you have hypochlorhydria, teas made from peppermint, ginseng, or ginger may help stimulate the flow of stomach acid. Try sipping a cup shortly before meals. An herbal-bitters tea made from gentian (the chief flavoring in angostura bitters) is another good way to stimulate stomach acid. To make this tea, boil one teaspoon of powdered gentian in half a cup of water for five minutes. Strain before drinking. Try gentian tea half an hour before meals; drink no more than two cups a day.

Juice therapy Bananas or banana juice can help soothe indigestion. For a smooth, creamy juice, combine one peeled banana with one cup of pear juice in the juicer or blender. Cantaloupe juice often helps settle indigestion. Try drinking a glass of fresh cantaloupe juice, or mix the cantaloupe juice half and half with pear juice. Have another glass an hour later if the first glass doesn't help. A cup of pear or peach juice, sipped slowly, may also help.

Hydrotherapy   A warm, wet compress on the abdomen is often all that is needed to relieve indigestion quickly. Activated charcoal as discussed above for heartburn is also useful for indigestion not accompanied by stomach gas. If you get indigestion often, try preventing it by drinking a glass of water mixed with one tablespoon of lemon juice or cider vinegar about an hour before meals.

Homeopathy   Homeopathic practitioners usually suggest carbo vegetabilis (carbo veg. or charcoal) 30c every ten to fifteen minutes for indigestion brought on by overeating or by eating fatty foods, especially if you also have bloating or gas; repeat up to seven times. Another remedy for indigestion with gas is lycopodium 6c, taken every three to four hours. Gas or bloating caused by nervousness may be helped by lycopodium 6c every half hour for up to ten doses. Indigestion caused by stress or nervousness may be helped by chamomilla 6c taken every three to four hours. Alternatively, try the tissue salt kali phosphoricum (kali phos. or potassium phosphate) 6x every three to four hours. Indigestion from overindulgence in alcohol is sometimes helped by nux vomica 6c taken every three to four hours.

Relaxation techniques   Indigestion in general and stomach gas in particular can be prevented by eating your meals in a relaxed, stress-free environment. Eat slowly and chew your food thoroughly. In addition, yoga exercises that tone the digestive system and abdominal area are often helpful.

Combined Treatments

Antacid/antigas medications and herbs To avoid the possible long-term effects of frequently using antacid/antigas medications, we often suggest trying herbal remedies first and moving on to the medications only if the herbal remedy doesn't provide relief.

Antacids and hydrotherapy The combination of antacids and a warm, wet compress often helps relieve indigestion symptoms faster than either treatment alone.

CHAPTER 3

Nausea and Vomiting

The word nausea comes from the Greek word for sea-sickness. In general, nausea refers to experiencing that awful abdominal feeling of queasiness, having an upset stomach, or being on the verge of vomiting. The unpleasant experience of vomiting occurs when your stomach contents are expelled through your mouth. As we'll discuss below, nausea and vomiting have many causes, including overindulgence in food or drink, gastroenteritis caused by minor illnesses or contaminated food, motion sickness, and morning sickness. Nausea and vomiting can also sometimes be caused by parasites or show up as side effects of prescription medications and cancer treatment. Gastritis and ulcers can also cause nausea and vomiting. (See chapter 4 on ulcers for more information.)

OVERINDULGENCE AND THE WRONG FOODS

Eating or drinking too much in general, or eating or drinking too much of a particular food or beverage, can lead to nausea and vomiting. Sometimes, however, even moderate amounts of a particular food will "disagree" with you and cause nausea. Greasy, fatty, or fried foods are the usual triggers; sometimes very spicy or very sweet foods cause the problem. Eating unaccustomed foods and spices may also cause nausea.

Traditional Treatments

Nausea and vomiting from overindulgence or eating something that disagrees with you are generally not serious. The discomfort usually passes within a few hours. Vomiting is often the best treatment for it, in fact, since it rids the stomach of the offending food or drink. If you feel extremely nauseous and on the brink of vomiting, don't fight the urge—simply let it all come up. It's unpleasant and possibly embarrassing, but you'll feel better. Don't try to induce vomiting, however.

Diet In cases of overindulgence, it's a little late to be thinking of diet. Prevent the problem next time by eating and drinking moderately and avoiding problem foods. In the meantime, eating a few dry crackers, a slice of dry toast, or some other bland, starchy food may help relieve your nausea. If you vomit, don't eat anything for an hour or so until your stomach settles; otherwise, anything you eat may come straight back up. After vomiting, rinse your mouth thoroughly with plain cool water to help get rid of the unpleasant taste. Slowly sip some plain cool water. Even a few sips will help wash corrosive stomach acid out of your esophagus and back into your stomach, which will help relieve the burning sensation in your esophagus. Once your stomach settles down again, try to replace the lost fluid by slowly sipping a large glass of cool water, mild herbal tea, or very diluted fruit juice (dilute juice by adding water). Avoid caffeineated or carbonated drinks of any sort—they will only make your nausea worse.

Self-help steps Avoid lying down or bending over until the nausea passes. If you feel nauseous from eating or drinking too much alcohol, a short walk in fresh air often helps.

Medication Nausea can often be relieved with pink bismuth (Pepto-Bismol). Some people find that antacids help. (See chapter 2 on heartburn and indigestion for more information about antacids.) Cola syrup, available at drugstores, often helps soothe an upset stomach; if you don't have any in your medicine cabinet, try some flat cola soda pop (carbonated cola will worsen the nausea). Over-the-counter phosphorated carbohydrate solutions such as Emetrol are helpful for relieving nausea. These products contain fructose, dextrose, and phosphoric acid. Avoid cola syrup and Emetrol if you should restrict your sugar intake for any reason.

Alternative Treatments

Acupressure The traditional acupressure points for nausea are pericardium points 5 and 6 (P5 and P6), which are located on the inside of both forearms. The P5 point is about two inches above the wrist; the P6 point is just next to it, a little closer to the wrist. Apply firm pressure with your thumb to the P5 point on your left arm for one minute, then repeat on the P6 point. Repeat again on the right side. This technique is particularly effective for making an attack of mild nausea pass quickly. If it doesn't work within ten minutes or so, try it again.

A traditional Japanese shiatzu remedy for nausea is to massage the calfs. Sit on the floor with your knees drawn up and your feet flat on the floor. Place your left thumb in the bend of your right knee; your left fingers will be resting on your shin. The shiatzu point you want to massage is on the outside of your right calf about where your left middle finger is pointing. Massage the point gently for ten to twenty seconds, then repeat twice more. Repeat three times on your left leg with your right hand.

Reflexology Gently massaging the stomach reflexes of the hands and feet can help relieve nausea. The stomach reflexes of each hand are found on the palm, in the area below the pads of the index and middle fingers. On each foot, the stomach reflexes are on the sole, in the area just below the large pad of the big toe. Repeat as needed.

Herbal therapy Numerous herbal remedies are traditionally recommended for nausea. Strong infusions of peppermint or chamomile tea (or a mix of the two) often help. Other herbs that are sometimes helpful are lemon balm and goldenseal. Weak tea without milk or sugar is also often helpful.

Ginger, a traditional Chinese remedy, is quite effective for relieving nausea. Tea made from freshly grated ginger root is most effective, although eating some candied ginger or even drinking some flat ginger ale can help. To make ginger tea, steep one teaspoon of freshly grated or finely chopped fresh ginger in one cup of boiling water for ten minutes. Strain before drinking. Tea bags containing dried ginger can be bought at health food stores; these work almost as well as making your own tea from fresh ginger. Capsules containing dried ground ginger are available at health food stores. Try taking one 500-milligram capsule instead of a cup of ginger tea. Additional cups of ginger tea or capsules can be taken as needed.

In traditional Ayurvedic medicine, nausea is treated with a tea made from cumin seeds. Steep one teaspoon of the seeds in a cup of boiling water for ten minutes. Strain before drinking.

Juice therapy   Fennel juice is useful for relieving discomfort from overeating. Juice only the stems, not the feathery tops of fresh fennel (the tops are very bitter). If you find the anise flavor too strong, add some carrot juice to the mixture. Slowly sipping a cup of pear or peach juice is another remedy that often helps.

Hydrotherapy   Another useful remedy for nausea from eating or drinking too much is activated charcoal, easily available at health food stores and well-stocked pharmacies. Mix two tablespoons of activated charcoal with one ounce of cool water in a twelve-ounce glass. When the mixture is well blended, slowly stir in enough water to fill the glass. Sip the mixture through a straw. Alternatively, swallow two activated charcoal tablets with a glass of water. Use activated charcoal only occasionally—frequent use can lead to impaired digestion and could interfere with any other medications you take.

Homeopathic remedies   There are several homeopathic remedies for nausea from overeating, especially if rich, fatty foods are the cause. Try pulsatilla 6c every ten to fifteen minutes until the discomfort passes; take no more than seven doses in total. Alternatively, try carbo vegetabilis 30c every ten to fifteen minutes until the discomfort passes; take no more than seven doses in total. Nux vomica 6c taken every ten to fifteen minutes is often very helpful, particularly if stress is adding to the problem. Repeat up to seven times. Ant. crud. 6c every three to four hours is often helpful if the nausea is more severe.

Combined Treatments

Diet and herbal remedies   Many patients benefit from eating bland foods and combating the nausea with herbal remedies. Drinking plenty of fluids, including mild herbal teas, is very beneficial if vomiting occurs.

Medications and herbal remedies If herbal remedies don't help relieve your nausea, try pink bismuth (Pepto-Bismol), an antacid, cola syrup, or Emetrol.

GASTROENTERITIS

Gastroenteritis is a minor illness, usually from a viral infection or contaminated food, that causes nausea and vomiting, along with diarrhea and perhaps a fever. Since there's often no way to tell exactly what is causing the illness, we just vaguely refer to "stomach bugs," "stomach or intestinal flus," or "twenty-four-hour viruses." Generally, such illnesses are minor, if uncomfortable, and clear up on their own within a day or two. (If you think your gastroenteritis is caused by contaminated food, see the discussion of food poisoning in chapter 8 later in this book.)

If your stomach flu continues for more than forty-eight hours without improving, if you are vomiting frequently for more than twenty-four hours or vomiting up blood or what looks like coffee grounds, or if your nausea and vomiting are accompanied by abdominal or chest pain or high fever, you may have a more serious problem. Call your doctor.

Vomiting and diarrhea can be serious problems for very young children, the elderly, or anyone with a chronic illness or a compromised immune system. Get medical attention quickly in such cases.

Traditional Treatments

Diet If you're having nausea and vomiting caused by gastroenteritis, you may not be very interested in eating. It's important to replace the fluids you lose, however, and you may feel hungry and thirsty in between periods of nausea. You'll feel better and recover faster if you stay well hydrated. Try sipping cool or warm (not icy or hot) beverages such as plain water, flat soda pop, diluted fruit juice, or mild herbal tea. Most people can keep down slightly salty clear liquids such as chicken broth or beef bouillon. Some people find sports beverages helpful; others find that sucking on ice pops (not ice cream) helps. Over the course of a day, try to take in six to eight cups of liquid or more. If you feel hungry, stick to plain carbohydrates such as crackers, dry toast, dry unsweetened breakfast cereal, rice, baked potatoes, plain oatmeal, and so on. Try nibbling on a peeled apple or a banana. Avoid milk products, protein, fibrous fruits and vegetables, and fatty or greasy foods.

Self-help steps You'll feel better and get over your illness faster if you stay home, rest, and drink plenty of fluids until the symptoms go away.

Medication Nausea can often be relieved with pink bismuth (Pepto-Bismol). Some people find that antacids help. (See chapter 2 on heartburn and indigestion for more information about antacids.) Cola syrup, available at drugstores, often helps soothe an upset stomach; if you don't have any in your medicine cabinet, try some flat cola soda pop. Over-the-counter phosphorated carbohydrate solutions such as Emetrol are helpful for relieving nausea. These products contain fructose, dextrose, and phosphoric acid. Avoid cola syrup and Emetrol if you should restrict your sugar intake for any reason.

Oral rehydration fluids such as Pedialyte are often helpful for babies and children suffering from gastroenteritis. These mixtures help prevent dangerous dehydration by restoring the water, potassium, and sodium and other electrolytes (body chemicals) that are lost as a result of frequent vomiting or diarrhea. Discuss oral rehydration fluids with your doctor before you use them.

Drugs that control nausea and vomiting are called antiemetics. If your nausea and vomiting are severe or continue for more than twenty-four to forty-eight hours without getting better, call your doctor. A prescription antiemetic may be needed.

Alternative Treatments

Acupressure The traditional acupressure points for nausea are pericardium points 5 and 6 (P5 and P6), which are located on the inside of both forearms. The P5 point is about two inches above the wrist; the P6 point is just next to it, a little closer to the wrist. Apply firm pressure with your thumb to the P5 point on your left arm for one minute, then repeat on the P6 point. Repeat again on the right side.

A traditional Japanese shiatzu remedy for nausea is to massage the calfs. Sit on the floor with your knees drawn up and your feet flat on the floor. Place your left thumb in the bend of your right knee; your left fingers will be resting on your shin. The shiatzu point you want to massage is on the outside of your right calf about where your left middle finger is pointing. Massage the point gently for ten to twenty seconds, then repeat twice more. Repeat three times on your left leg with your right hand.

Reflexology Gently massaging the stomach reflexes of the hands and feet can help relieve nausea. The stomach reflexes of your hand are found on the palm, in the area below the pads of the index and middle fingers. On your feet, the stomach reflexes are on the soles, in the area just below the large pads of the big toes. Repeat as needed.

Herbal therapy Peppermint or chamomile tea (or a mixture of the two) often helps relieve nausea. Ginger, a traditional Chinese remedy, is quite effective. Tea made from freshly grated ginger root is most effective, although eating some candied ginger or even drinking some flat ginger ale (ginger ale that has lost its fizz) can help. To make ginger tea, steep one teaspoon of freshly grated or finely chopped fresh ginger in one cup of boiling water for ten minutes. Strain before drinking. Capsules containing dried ground ginger are available at health food stores. If you have been vomiting, however, you may have trouble keeping ginger down. If possible, take the tea or capsules when you first start to feel nauseous—this may help keep you from throwing up.

In traditional Ayurvedic medicine, nausea is treated with a tea made from cumin seeds. Steep one teaspoon of the seeds in a cup of boiling water for ten minutes. Strain before drinking.

Homeopathic remedies Homeopaths suggest several different remedies for nausea from gastroenteritis. The remedy most often recommended is ipecac 6c, taken every half hour for up to seven doses. For severe nausea, pulsatilla 6c can be taken every fifteen minutes for up to ten doses; in less severe cases, take pulsatilla hourly for up to ten doses. If the nausea is accompanied by diarrhea, try arsen. alb. 6c hourly for up to ten doses. If you feel exhausted from vomiting, try china 6c every half hour up to seven doses.

Combined Treatments
Diet and herbal remedies   Eat bland foods and fight the nausea with herbal remedies. Drinking plenty of fluids, including mild herbal teas, is very beneficial if vomiting occurs.

Medications and herbal remedies   If herbal remedies don't help relieve your nausea, try pink bismuth (Pepto-Bismol), an antacid, cola syrup, or Emetrol.

MOTION SICKNESS

Many patients say that of all the unpleasant forms of nausea, motion sickness is the worst. The extreme nausea and vomiting of motion sickness, accompanied by dizziness, headache, cold sweats, and excess salivation, are enough to ruin any outing and make long trips by car, train, plane, or boat a misery. Motion sickness is caused by constant, unpredictable movement, such as the rocking of a small boat on rough water. The motion affects the inner ear, causing the nausea and other symptoms. Once the movement stops, motion sickness goes away almost at once.

For unknown reasons, some people are much more susceptible to motion sickness than others. One of our patients got motion sickness from the high-speed elevator in his office tower. The problem sometimes lessens or goes away with age. Young children often get carsick, for example, and "grow out of it" as they get older. Motion sickness may also go away as people get used to the movement. Travelers on cruise ships often experience mild seasickness during the first day or two, and then get over it. Even experienced sailors, however, will get seasick in very rough conditions.

Traditional Treatments

Diet   What you eat can do a lot to help prevent motion sickness or reduce the severity of the symptoms. Being hungry can actually make you more likely to get motion sickness, so eat a small, simple meal one to two hours before the trip begins. Stick to easily digested, bland carbohydrates such as plain bread, crackers, baked potatoes, rice, and the like. Apples, bananas, and well-steamed vegetables are also good choices. Avoid greasy or fatty foods, large amounts of protein, spicy foods, and milk products. While traveling, stay with the same simple foods. Before and during the trip, avoid caffeine, milk, carbonated beverages, acidic fruit juices, and alcohol in any form.

Self-help steps   You can prevent or relieve motion sickness with some simple measures. Get plenty of fresh air during your trip—seat yourself near an open window or aim the fresh-air vent of your airplane seat toward you. Avoid unpleasant smells such as cooking odors, exhaust fumes, and tobacco smoke. Face forward in the direction of the vehicle's motion. Being able to see the horizon helps many people, so stay on deck on a boat or sit in the front seat of a car. Trying to focus on reading materials, playing cards, and the like will only make your motion sickness worse. Sit quietly instead.

Drugs   Several over-the-counter drugs can help prevent or treat motion sickness, especially if taken before the start of the trip. Well-known brands include Dramamine (dimenhydrinate) and Bonine (meclizine hydrochloride); their generic equivalents are less expensive and work just as well, though fewer doses of Bonine are needed. These drugs are safe and effective, but they can cause drowsiness. Do not take them with any other tranquilizer or sedative, and do not drink alcohol. Do not drive or perform any other action that requires concentration and good responses while taking these drugs. Do not take these drugs if you have asthma, glaucoma, lung disease, or prostate problems.

If you are planning a trip and know you are likely to get motion sickness, your doctor may prescribe prescription-strength dimenhydrinate (Dramamine). If you are going on a long trip such as a cruise, your doctor may prescribe scopalamine in the form of a long-lasting skin patch (Transderm Scōp). Scopalamine is very effective for the prevention and treatment of motion sickness, especially in this form. The unobtrusive, painless patch is placed on the hairless skin behind your ear and releases the scopalamine at a steady rate over a three-day period. Put the patch on several hours before the trip begins; it is safe to apply a new patch when the original patch is used up. Wash your hands thoroughly immediately after putting on the patch; if scopalamine from the patch gets on your fingers and is transferred to your eyes, it will cause you to have temporary blurred vision and pupil dilation (widening).

Scopalamine is a potent drug and should not be used by children, the elderly, or by anyone who has glaucoma. It may cause drowsiness and confusion, so don't drive a vehicle or do anything that requires mental alertness while you are taking it. While wearing the patch and even for a few days after, your eyes may be somewhat more sensitive to light than usual. To counteract this effect, wear sunglasses. It's also possible that one pupil will appear slightly larger than the other. This effect is harmless and will go away after you stop wearing the patch.

Alternative Treatments

Acupressure   Acupressure is an excellent way to prevent and relieve motion sickness. As with other forms of nausea, the traditional acupressure points are pericardium points 5 and 6 (P5 and P6), which are located on the inside of both forearms. The P5 point is about two inches above the wrist; the P6 point is just next to it, a little closer to the wrist. Applying firm pressure to these points may briefly relieve the symptoms—it worked very well for the patient who got sick in elevators. Motion sickness will continue as long the motion does, however, so you'll probably need to apply constant pressure. An acupressure wrist band is the most convenient way to do this; this is an inexpensive device, generally made from an elastic band that has a small ball attached. The ball is positioned over the acupressure point on the wrist and applies a steady pressure. Acupressure bands are easily available in drugstores and health food stores. They work best if you put one on each wrist before the motion begins.

Herbal therapy   Powdered ginger in capsules is a very effective herbal remedy for motion sickness. Ginger capsules are sold in health food stores. Take one or two 500-milligram capsules half an hour before your trip begins; if you get severe motion sickness, you may need to take up to four capsules before the trip starts. If capsules aren't available, try eating candied ginger or drinking ginger tea (see the section on overindulgence above for more information). Even flat ginger ale may help. Take additional capsules during your trip as needed, preferably at the first hint of nausea.

Homeopathic remedies   To help prevent the onset of motion sickness, homeopaths often suggest tabacum 6c every fifteen minutes, starting one hour before you begin your trip. Take no more than ten doses. Nux vomica 6c, taken every fifteen minutes, may also be effective. Start one hour before you begin your trip; take no more than ten doses. Petroleum 6c, taken every half hour, may help. Start one hour before you begin your trip; take no more than seven doses. Cocculus 6c, taken every three to four hours, may also help prevent motion sickness. Take the dose one hour before you begin your trip. Once motion sickness has begun, the remedies above may still help relieve it. Alternatively, try the most commonly used homeopathic remedy for nausea: ipecac 6c, taken every fifteen minutes for up to ten doses.

Relaxation techniques   Deep-breathing techniques sometimes help ward off motion sickness. If you start to feel nauseous, sit upright, facing forward. Breathe in slowly and deeply through your nose, pulling the air deep into your lungs. Breathe out again slowly and deeply through your nose, exhaling as much as possible. Repeat until the nausea passes.

Combined Treatments

Diet, self-help steps, acupressure, and ginger   Because motion-sickness drugs can cause unpleasant side effects, I prefer to recommend them only for severe cases. If you know you are likely to get motion sickness, a combination of diet and self-help steps, along with acupressure wrist bands and ginger capsules, may prevent the problem completely and will probably reduce the discomfort sharply if you do get sick.

Self-help, acupressure, and relaxation techniques

Sometimes motion sickness strikes unexpectedly. Self-help steps, combined with acupressure and relaxation techniques, may help relieve the symptoms.

MORNING SICKNESS

Almost every pregnant woman experiences at least some morning sickness. The nausea, vomiting, and fatigue of morning sickness are usually worst during the first three months of pregnancy, although some unfortunate women have the symptoms until the day the baby is delivered, while a lucky few don't really get morning sickness at all.

Although scientists are still researching the causes of morning sickness, many today feel that the normal hormonal changes of pregnancy are the basic cause. Specifically, they think the human hormone chorionic gonadotropin (HCG), the same hormone that is detected by pregnancy tests, is the main trigger. Because HCG levels are at their highest during the first three months of pregnancy, this would help explain why morning sickness is also usually worst during that period. As HCG levels drop after the first trimester, many women find that their morning sickness improves or even goes away completely. Morning sickness has nothing to do with stress or any ambivalent feelings women may have about being pregnant.

Severe morning sickness with frequent vomiting, or prolonged nausea that doesn't go away over the course of the day, may indicate a more serious problem. If your morning sickness is very bad or suddenly becomes worse, call your doctor.

Traditional Treatments

Diet   Morning sickness may be perfectly normal, but it occurs just at the time when good nutrition is very important both for the mother-to-be and her unborn baby. The challenge is to find ways to keep eating well at a time when the mere thought of food can bring on the dreaded symptoms.

One trick that often works very well is to eat some plain carbohydrates immediately after waking in the morning, even before getting out of bed. Plain unsalted crackers or unsweetened breakfast cereal are good choices. The bland food seems to reduce the nausea and reduce vomiting, although it may not relieve the symptoms completely. Keep some of these foods handy to nibble if the nausea returns during the day.

You'll probably feel better during the day if you have some food in your stomach. Try to eat small, nutritious meals or snacks every couple of hours, or whenever you feel hungry or think you can keep food down. Avoid large meals and greasy, fatty, or very rich foods such as cream sauces. Spicy foods, acidic foods, and foods with strong odors are likely to worsen your morning sickness. Try to avoid foods that you already know upset your digestion. Stick to plain carbohydrates, such as baked potatoes, toast, rice, and pasta, fresh fruits and vegetables, flavored gelatin, cottage cheese, and simply prepared foods such as baked chicken. Don't be limited by this list, however—feel free to eat whatever appeals to you whenever you like.

Be sure to drink plenty of liquids to replace the fluids you lose. Plain water, diluted fruit juice, ice pops, mild herbal teas, and simple broths or soups are all good choices. Do not drink alcohol or beverages containing caffeine.

Self-help steps   Because pregnant women have a heightened sense of smell, unpleasant aromas or strong smells often trigger morning sickness. The only solution is to try to avoid smells or get away from them quickly into fresh air. The smell of food or cooking is a very common trigger. At such times, food preparation is out of the question—if possible, get someone else to do the shopping and cooking.

Try not to eat for at least two hours before going to sleep—this may help reduce nighttime heartburn and morning nausea.

Fatigue is often a symptom of morning sickness. If you feel very fatigued, don't force yourself to keep going. Rest quietly or take a nap instead. Avoid stimulating caffeine beverages such as coffee, tea, hot chocolate, cola, and some soft drinks.

Medication   Physicians are extremely reluctant to suggest any sort of drug for a pregnant woman. Discuss the use of nonprescription antacids or other over-the-counter drugs for heartburn and nausea with your doctor before you try them. In very severe cases of morning sickness, prescription drugs may be recommended.

Alternative Treatments

Acupressure   Acupressure often works well to relieve the nausea of morning sickness. The traditional acupressure points for nausea are pericardium points 5 and 6 (P5 and P6), which are located on the inside of both forearms. The P5 point is about two inches above the wrist; the P6 point is just next to it, a little closer to the wrist.

Apply firm pressure with your thumb to the P5 point on your left arm for one minute, then repeat on the P6 point. Repeat again on the right side. This technique is particularly effective for making an attack of mild nausea pass quickly. Repeat as needed.

An acupressure wrist band may help prevent bouts of morning sickness throughout the day. An inexpensive device, this is generally made from an elastic band that has a small ball attached; the ball is positioned over the acupressure point on the wrist and applies a steady pressure. Try wearing one on each wrist; put them on as soon as you wake up in the morning.

A traditional Japanese shiatzu remedy for nausea is to massage the calfs. Sit on the floor with your knees drawn up and your feet flat on the floor. Place your left thumb in the bend of your right knee; your left fingers will be resting on your shin. The shiatzu point you want to massage is on the outside of your right calf about where your left middle finger is pointing. Massage the point gently for ten to twenty seconds, then repeat twice more. Repeat three times on your left leg with your right hand.

Herbal therapy   Ginger, a traditional Chinese herbal remedy for nausea, helps many women with morning sickness. Some women find that swallowing two 500-milligram ginger capsules as soon as they wake up helps reduce morning sickness. During the day, try drinking some ginger tea or taking one or two additional 500-milligram capsules of powdered ginger when nausea strikes. To make ginger tea, steep one teaspoon of freshly grated or finely chopped fresh ginger in one cup of boiling water for ten minutes. Strain before drinking. Tea bags containing dried ginger can be bought at health food stores; these work almost as well as making your own tea from fresh ginger. Capsules containing dried, ground ginger are available at health food stores.

Mild herbal teas such as peppermint and chamomile can help relieve the nausea of morning sickness and help restore fluids after vomiting. Black raspberry leaf tea is a traditional herbal remedy. Be sure to purchase exactly that at the health food store—don't get raspberry-flavored black tea instead.

Homeopathic remedies   Homeopathic practitioners generally suggest nux vomica 6c every two hours for morning sickness. Use it for no more than three days. Pulsatilla 6c every two hours is suggested for morning sickness that is worse in the evening; take it for no more than three days. Morning sickness that causes general nausea all day long may be helped by ipecac 6c taken every two hours; take it for no more than three days. Other homeopathic remedies that sometimes help include tabacum 6c taken every three to four hours and sepia 6c, taken every three to four hours. Sepia is said to be particularly helpful if the smell of food has brought on the nausea.

Relaxation techniques   Deep-breathing exercises as discussed above in the section on motion sickness can often relieve a wave of nausea.

Combined Treatments
Diet, acupressure, and herbal treatments   By eating carefully and using acupressure and herbal remedies, you can do a lot to relieve the worst symptoms of morning sickness. Unfortunately, the symptoms will probably not go away entirely, especially during the first three months of your pregnancy. To a degree, you will probably just have to wait out your morning sickness.

CHAPTER 4

Peptic Ulcer Disease

Until very recently, peptic ulcers were among the most frustrating of ailments, for both the patient and the health care provider. Diet, drugs, alternative therapies, and even surgery usually helped, but the relapse rate was high and very few patients were ever fully cured. Our lack of good treatments had a high cost: peptic ulcer disease will affect about 10 percent of all Americans—about 25 million people—during their lifetime.

Fortunately, our understanding of peptic ulcer disease has changed radically in just the past few years. We now know its cause and we now know how to cure it—quickly, easily, and for good.

A peptic ulcer is a painful, craterlike sore in the mucous membrane lining your stomach or your duodenum. Peptic ulcers in the stomach are called gastric ulcers; peptic ulcers in the duodenum are called duodenal ulcers. Gastritis is an inflammation of the mucous membrane that lines your stomach. Almost all of us get occasional gastritis from overeating, eating a food that "disagrees" with us, or drinking too much alcohol, but we do not all have peptic ulcer disease. Chronic gastritis, however, is characterized by frequent severe stomach pain and nausea not related to excess food or drink. People with chronic gastritis are more likely to develop peptic ulcers.

Gastric ulcers are often fairly large—an inch or more in diameter. Duodenal ulcers tend to be smaller, usually less than half an inch in diameter. No matter what the size or location of the ulcer, the principal symptom is severe pain. Peptic ulcers cause a burning, gnawing pain, generally across the upper part of the abdomen and sometimes into the chest. The pain usually lasts for anywhere from thirty minutes to several hours; it is often relieved somewhat by eating. The pain may go away for short periods, but it almost always comes back. The pain of a duodenal ulcer is just as intense, but it tends to be more localized in a small area of the upper abdomen. Duodenal ulcer pain is more likely to occur predictably several hours after a meal. A related problem, nonulcer dyspepsia, causes abdominal pain very similar to that of an ulcer, even though none actually exists. The pain tends to occur early in the morning and is often in the same place in the abdomen. Eating or taking an antacid often relieves the symptoms.

For decades, physicians believed that ulcers were caused by excess stomach acid that ate through the protective mucous lining of the stomach or duodenum and attacked the underlying muscle. Stress was believed to cause the excess acid, which in turn caused the craterlike ulcer sore. Medical treatment of a peptic ulcer usually meant a recommendation of bland foods and dairy products, which were believed to neutralize the acid, and attempts, through drugs, psychotherapy, and others means, to reduce the patient's stress level. Chronic gastritis was also attributed to excess acid and stress; the treatment was usually similar.

Unfortunately, none of the treatments worked very well or for very long. Some actually made the ulcer worse. Dairy products, especially milk and cream, contain calcium, which stimulates the stomach to produce *more* acid. A bland diet helped some ulcer patients, while others got sicker eating the same foods. It was also increasingly clear that excess stomach acid really didn't have much to do with ulcers, since some people who produced almost no acid still got ulcers, while others who produced large amounts of acid never had any symptoms at all. The stress connection was even harder to prove. Many people who led happy, apparently stress-free lives got ulcers, while others who led miserable, very high-stress lives never did. And even when high-stress individuals with ulcers learned to slow down their lives and relax, their ulcers persisted. Liquid antacids and some dietary changes did help many people with ulcers, but the problem never really went away.

Ulcer and chronic gastritis treatment improved greatly in the late 1970s, when H_2 blockers such as Tagamet, Axid, and Zantac, which sharply reduce the production of stomach acid, were introduced. Ulcer treatment improved even more in 1989, when Prilosec (omeprazole) was introduced. Prilosec turns off stomach acid production completely. As long as the patient took one of these drugs, the ulcers remained under control. When the drug was stopped, the ulcers almost always returned. To prevent recurrence, the patient needed to take prescription-strength doses essentially for life. By one 1994 estimate, the cost of the drugs over fifteen years was $11,500.

In recent years, the diagnosis and treatment of peptic ulcers and gastritis has changed drastically for the better. This is due to the discovery, by Dr. Barry Marshall in

Perth, Australia, that a bacterium called *Helicobacter pylori* is the cause of almost all peptic ulcer disease. In 1985, Dr. Marshall proved that *H. pylori* causes the disease when he himself deliberately ingested a dose of the bacteria. He didn't get an ulcer, but he did develop a severe case of gastritis, which he then cured with standard antibiotics. Further research confirmed his findings. Almost all people who suffer from peptic ulcers or chronic gastritis are infected with the *H. pylori* bacterium, a spiral-shaped organism that manages to survive in the highly acidic environment of the stomach. Studies also strongly suggest that most people with gastric cancer are infected with the bacterium. In 1994, the National Institutes of Health adopted new protocols for physicians that recommend eradicating the bacterium as the primary method for treating ulcers.

The unmistakable, severe gnawing or burning pain in the upper part of the abdomen is the chief symptom of a peptic ulcer or chronic gastritis. The pain is most likely to occur one to two hours after you eat, since stomach acid levels will be high then. Food temporarily soaks up some of your stomach acid, so eating ("feeding your ulcer") may briefly relieve the pain; the pain comes back as soon as the food leaves your stomach. Nonprescription antacids or H_2 blockers such as Zantac may also briefly help the pain. Other symptoms of an ulcer may include nausea, vomiting, and loss of appetite.

An ulcer is so painful that it will probably send you to your doctor quickly. Don't delay or treat yourself with antacids if you think you have an ulcer or chronic gastritis. The discomfort will only get worse, and the problem will not just go away. If you vomit blood or something that looks like coffee grounds, or if you have black, tarry stools, your ulcer may be bleeding—even though you may not be having any pain. Get medical attention at once!

To confirm the presence of an ulcer, your doctor will insert a thin, flexible, lighted tube called an endoscope down your esophagus and into your stomach. While it would be untrue to say the endoscopy experience is pleasant, there is really very little discomfort (your doctor will spray a local anesthetic on the back of your throat), and the procedure is over quickly. Sometimes the doctor will use the endoscope to take a tiny tissue sample of the ulcerated area.

To confirm the presence of the *Helicobacter pylori* bacterium, your doctor may do a simple, inexpensive, very accurate blood test. A drawback to this is that the blood test does not distinguish between an active infection and a past infection. An even faster method for determining an active infection is a breath test that measures the amount of urease, a metabolic waste product of *H. pylori*, in your exhaled breath. Until recently, this test required a fairly elaborate piece of equipment and was performed mostly at large medical centers. In late 1996, however, the Food and Drug Administration (FDA) approved a simpler breath test that can be done in the doctor's office; results are available in a day or two.

Even if your doctor suspects nonulcer dyspepsia and doesn't see an ulcer during endoscopic examination, he or she will probably do a blood test for *H. pylori* just to make sure. If *H. pylori* is present, the treatment will be the same as for ulcers. If the bacteria are not present, the treatment is essentially the same as that for mild heartburn: antacids or over-the-counter H_2 blockers, combined with dietary and self-help steps and whatever alternative treatments are effective for you. (See chapter 2 on heartburn for more information.)

Occasionally people who take large doses of nonsteroidal anti-inflammatory drugs (NSAIDs), such as aspirin, ibuprofen, prescription-strength arthritis medications, steroids, and some other prescription drugs develop gastric erosion, a small area of inflammation in the stomach that may be painful or may bleed. Sometimes these patients develop a full-fledged ulcer. The drug is usually blamed, but in a surprisingly large number of cases the patient is infected with *H. pylori*. If you think a drug you are taking is causing severe heartburn or ulcerlike pain, call your doctor. You may be able to change the dosage or the medication or take antacids to relieve the symptoms. Your doctor may also wish to test for *H. pylori*.

Traditional Treatments

Usually health care providers begin with the simplest treatments and move on to drugs and other treatments only if necessary. In the case of ulcers, however, drug treatment should begin as soon as the ulcer is diagnosed. Diet and stress reduction are now considered far less important in ulcer treatment, although they still play a role.

Drugs   Right now, the best and most effective treatment for peptic ulcer disease is a combination of two drugs. The antibiotic amoxicillin (Amoxil, Polymox, Trimox, Wymox, or the generic equivalent) is given to kill the *H. pylori* bacteria; omeprazole (Prilosec) is used to stop stomach acid production, which relieves the pain and allows the ulcer to heal. This double treatment is inexpensive, very effective, and easy to follow, since the drugs are usually taken just twice a day for only two weeks. If you still have pain from your ulcer after the antibiotic treatment is complete, your doctor may recommend that you continue to take Prilosec or an H$_2$ blocker for several more weeks until the ulcer has healed completely.

If you are allergic to amaxicillin, which is a type of penicillin, your doctor may prescribe a triple combination of drugs: pink bismuth (Pepto Bismol), the antibiotics metronidazole (Flagyl or the generic equivalent) or tetracycline, and ranitidine (Zantac). The pink bismuth fights the bacteria, as do the antibiotics, while the Zantac or its equivalent reduces stomach acid. Triple-combination therapy can get complicated to follow, however, and you are also more likely to have mild side effects, such as diarrhea.

Careful studies have shown that either treatment is quite likely to eradicate the *H. pylori* bacteria completely. Your ulcer will probably heal completely within ten weeks, and you will probably not have a recurrence. After you've completed the drug treatment, your doctor will do another test to confirm that the bacteria have been killed off completely. Breath tests are somewhat more effective than blood tests for determining this, although both tests are very accurate. In about 10 to 15 percent of all cases, drug treatment does not completely eradicate the bacteria. In such cases, you may need to repeat the treatment to avoid a recurrence later on.

Amoxicillin can be taken on a full or empty stomach. However, if your treatment includes the antibiotic tetracycline, take the medicine on an empty stomach with a full glass of water or as directed by your doctor. Avoid eating or drinking dairy products for one to two hours before and after taking tetracycline; these foods can reduce the drug's effectiveness.

If you regularly take any other drugs, including nonprescription medications such as aspirin or ibuprofen (Advil), be sure to tell your doctor before starting drug therapy for your ulcer.

Diet While you are taking drugs to treat your ulcer, your diet can help make the treatment more effective; it can also reduce the discomfort. There's no reason to follow the traditional bland ulcer diet, but you might want to temporarily avoid very spicy, fatty, or acidic foods. Also avoid any foods that you already know tend to upset your digestion. Because protein stimulates the stomach to produce acid, some patients find that they feel better if they cut back on meat for the first couple of weeks of treatment. Otherwise, the usual diet will be fine.

If eating has helped relieve your ulcer pain in the past, try eating six small meals spread evenly across the day instead of three larger meals. Avoid caffeine, alcohol, and carbonated beverages. Even decaf coffee may cause discomfort, so cut back or give it up until your ulcer is better.

Self-help steps Taking your medicine as directed, for the full length of the treatment, is the most important self-help step you can take. Most people start to feel a lot better as soon as they begin taking Prilosec or an H_2 blocker and can quickly return to their normal activities while treatment continues.

Smoking will make your ulcer pain worse, could interfere with your drug treatment, and may even cause you to develop new ulcers. If you smoke, stop.

Surgery At one time, surgery to remove the part of the stomach or small intestine affected by the ulcer was a last-resort treatment for very severe or intractable cases—and even then the ulcers sometimes came back.

Today that operation has become so uncommon that some younger surgeons have never even learned how to do it. Sometimes, however, an untreated ulcer can become so deep that it perforates through or erodes the wall of the stomach or small intestine. A perforated ulcer is acutely painful and requires emergency medical care; surgery may be needed to repair the hole.

Complementary Treatments

Because ulcers are so common and, until recently, didn't respond well to traditional medical treatment, there are many alternative therapies. In the past, some of these, such as licorice (DGL) capsules made from licorice roots, often worked just as well as the available medical treatment. Today, however, antibiotic treatment is much more effective than any alternative treatment—not only for relieving the immediate discomfort of the ulcer but for curing the infection completely, healing the ulcer completely, and reducing the chance of recurrence to practically nothing. The alternative treatments discussed below should therefore be considered as supplements to, not replacements for, antibiotic treatment. Discuss them with your physician before you try them.

Reflexology   Gently massaging the stomach reflexes of the hands and feet can help relieve ulcer symptoms. The stomach reflexes of each hand are found on the palm, in the area below the pads of the index and middle fingers. On each foot, the stomach reflexes are on the sole, in the area just below the large pad of the big toe. Some reflexologists believe that massaging the diaphragm and solar plexus reflex points of the hands and feet also helps relieve ulcer discomfort. These points overlap on each hand in the palm, just below the pad of the middle finger.

They also overlap on the sole just below the ball of the foot.

Herbal therapy   Herbal remedies for ulcers abound. Some do help relieve the discomfort of an ulcer, but none will cure it or keep it from coming back. Use these remedies only after discussing them with your doctor.

Licorice root *(Glycyrrhiza glabra)* is a traditional herbal treatment that is said to act as a demulcent, or herb that soothes the mucous membranes. It can be taken as a tea made from a teaspoonful of the licorice root (easily available at health food stores) steeped in half a cup of water for five minutes. Strain before drinking; take half a cup three times a day after meals. Stop using licorice root if you notice any swelling in your face, hands, or feet, and don't use it for longer than four weeks. Deglycyrrhizinated licorice (DGL), in the form of capsules, is more convenient, however, and less likely to cause side effects. Take two capsules four times daily.

Licorice root and DGL can cause you to retain fluids. Don't use either if you have high blood pressure, heart disease, liver disease, or diabetes.

Marshmallow root is also said to be soothing to the mucous membranes. To make a decoction from this herb, combine one teaspoonful of the marshmallow root with one cup of water and simmer for fifteen minutes. Let cool and strain before drinking. Take no more than three cups a day after meals.

Another soothing demulcent is slippery elm bark. To make slippery elm bark tea, combine one teaspoon of the bark in two cups of water for twenty minutes. Let cool and strain before drinking. Drink no more than four cups a day. Slippery elm bark is also available in convenient capsules. Take two to four capsules daily.

Gentian and strong chamomile tea are traditional herbal remedies that can be helpful. Other remedies that are sometimes recommended by herbalists include alfalfa (juice or tablets), red clover flowers, and kelp, but these herbs are unlikely to provide any relief.

In traditional Chinese medicine, ginger and ginseng are often recommended for ulcers. Ginger is particularly effective for some patients, perhaps because it reduces the production of stomach acid. To make ginger tea, steep one teaspoon of freshly grated or finely chopped fresh ginger in one cup of boiling water for ten minutes. Strain before drinking. Tea bags containing dried ginger can be bought at health food stores; these work almost as well as making your own tea from fresh ginger. Capsules containing dried ground ginger are also available at health food stores. Try taking one 500-milligram capsule instead of a cup of ginger tea. Ginseng is usually taken as a tea made from the powdered root. To prepare ginseng tea, steep one to three teaspoons of ginseng in one cup of boiling water for ten minutes, stirring occasionally. Stir before drinking. Ginseng tablets and capsules are available in various dosages. Herbalists generally suggest daily doses ranging from 500 milligrams to two grams.

Traditional Ayurvedic medicine recommends aloe vera gel for treating ulcers. The usual dose is one to two teaspoons three times a day. Aloe vera gel has a very bitter flavor, so try mixing it with honey. Be very careful about the product you purchase. Make sure it is an aloe vera gel meant for internal use for stomach problems, and not one for external use or for use as a laxative.

Vitamin and mineral supplements Iron supplements can irritate the stomach and small intestine. Avoid them while your ulcer is healing. Your ulcer may heal faster if you take some extra vitamins and minerals, such as daily supplements of 10,000 IU of vitamin A, 100 milligrams of B complex vitamins, and 1,000 milligrams of buffered vitamin C. Zinc picolinate also aids healing; the recommended dose is 50 milligrams a day.

Dietary supplements Your stomach and intestines need the amino acid glutamine as a fuel source and for healing. Supplemental glutamine has helped many of our ulcer patients heal faster. We suggest taking one 500-milligram glutamine capsule four times a day for six to ten weeks or until the ulcer has healed. If you prefer, try substituting eight ounces of fresh cabbage juice for one or two of the glutamine capsules.

Rice bran oil, also called gamma oryzanol, is an ulcer treatment that has been widely used in Japan. It is sold in capsules in health food stores. Some people find that taking one capsule three times a day helps relieve their ulcer symptoms. Rice bran oil may also help the ulcer heal faster.

Some patients find that the antibiotic part of their ulcer treatment upsets their digestion and gives them mild diarrhea. This occurs because the antibiotics kill not only the harmful *H. pylori* bacteria but also some of the beneficial bacteria found in the intestines. To help restore the proper balance of bacteria after you have stopped taking the antibiotics, try to avoid refined sugar in any form, eat a diet low in fat and high in complex carbohydrates, and have a daily six-ounce serving of a fermented dairy product such as unflavored live-culture yogurt (available in health food stores). If your digestion doesn't seem to return to normal after a few weeks, you may need to take additional dietary measures (see the discussion of dysbiosis in chapter 6 for detailed information).

Juice therapy   Some patients report that drinking fresh cabbage juice helps their symptoms. This may work because cabbage juice is high in glutamine (see the discussion of dietary supplements above for more information). Cabbage juice is also high in sulfur compounds, which may have a healing effect on the stomach lining. Try sipping a cup of fresh cabbage juice if ulcer symptoms occur. If the cabbage taste is too strong, try diluting the juice with an equal amount of some other green juice, such as celery or parsley.

Homeopathy   The homeopathic remedy graphites 6c, taken every ten to fifteen minutes for up to seven doses, may help relieve mild ulcer discomfort.

Relaxation techniques   Stress does not cause ulcers, but it can slow the healing process. Try to slow down a little during your drug therapy and for a few weeks after it is over to help your ulcer heal as quickly as possible.

Combined Treatments

Drugs, vitamin and mineral supplements, and dietary supplements   The only cure for ulcers is drug treatment to eliminate the *H. pylori* bacteria. The ulcer may heal faster if you take vitamin and mineral supplements along with the amino acid glutamine. Fermented dairy products may help restore a good balance of bacteria in your intestines once the antibiotic treatment is complete.

CHAPTER 5

Food Allergies and Sensitivities

Food allergies are a somewhat controversial topic among health care practitioners. Some believe that true food allergies are rare, affecting no more than 1 percent of the population. Others believe that many people—perhaps more than half the population—suffer from negative responses to the foods they eat and that food allergies are responsible for a wide range of symptoms. In this chapter, we'll discuss food allergies and intolerances, both in general and with specific reference to lactose intolerance (the inability to digest milk) and celiac disease, which is also called sprue (the inability to digest gluten).

FOOD ALLERGIES

In the narrow medical definition, a food allergy occurs when something that most people can ingest without harm causes your body's immune system to react immediately and adversely. The allergic reaction can be anything from a mild case of hives to anaphylactic shock, but it always occurs predictably soon after you consume the offending food. Today the word allergy is often used more broadly to mean any sort of negative response, immediate or delayed, to something you eat or drink. For the sake of accuracy in both diagnosis and treatment, we have to distinguish between these two usages of the word. If the response involves the immune system, it is a true food allergy (also sometimes called atopic allergy). If the response does not involve the immune system, it is a food intolerance or sensitivity. There is an in-between category of reactions that is caused by natural substances in foods and by food additives. Although these are not always true allergic reactions, the symptoms are similar.

In this section, we'll discuss true food allergies and reactions to chemicals in food. We'll discuss food intolerances in the section following this one. If you think you might have a food allergy, please be sure to read both sections.

Traditional Treatments

No one really knows why some people have an immune-system response to a particular food. The most likely explanation is that for unknown reasons some immune systems mistake a protein in the food for an invading protein. When specialized immune system cells called type IgE antibodies detect the food protein, they go on the rampage, releasing chemical messengers that in turn trigger other cells to release chemicals such as cytokines, leukotrienes, and histamines. These substances trigger the symptoms of the allergic response. Food allergies generally cause respiratory or skin symptoms: a runny nose, sneezing, tearing eyes, itching, hives, skin rashes, flushing, wheeziness, or an asthma attack. Less common symptoms of food allergies include swelling around the mouth or in the throat, gas, bloating, nausea and vomiting, and cramps and diarrhea.

In very severe cases, anaphylactic shock can occur: severe itching or hives, swelling of the throat, difficulty breathing, and a sudden, severe drop in blood pressure. This is a medical emergency that requires immediate treatment. Fortunately, anaphylactic reactions are rare.

Food allergies are most common in children under the age of six—more than 5 percent of all children have them. Most children eventually grow out of them, but for some, food allergies will persist throughout their lives to some extent. Some babies and young children are allergic to cow's milk. This is a true allergy that requires medical diagnosis and is usually treated by switching the child to a soy formula. As we'll discuss below, a milk allergy is not the same thing as lactose intolerance. Babies and children are also more likely to be allergic to eggs and wheat. If you suspect food allergies in your child, see your pediatrician immediately.

Most adults develop a food allergy suddenly, often after eating the allergic food harmlessly for years. Researchers still don't know why this happens. Once you've developed the allergy, you'll have it for life.

Food allergy symptoms generally occur very soon after you have eaten the offending food, so you will probably be able to quickly pinpoint the source of the reaction. To confirm the food allergy and detect any others, your doctor will probably use the RAST (radioallergosorbent test) or the more sensitive ELISA (enzyme-linked immunoserological assay) blood test.

Diet   The best treatment for a food allergy is complete avoidance. Once you have been sensitized, even a small amount of the allergic food will cause a reaction—and the reaction is likely to be more severe each time you are exposed. Interestingly, some people find that their food reactions are tied to their other allergic reactions. For example, many people who are allergic to ragweed and other airborne pollens are also allergic to melons such as cantaloupe, honeydew, and watermelon and to herbs such as goldenseal and chamomile. These people may react to the foods, however, only during ragweed season. Even so, the best course is not to take chances: if you know you are allergic to a food, don't eat it.

If you have a food allergy, it is most likely to be to nuts, peanuts and other legumes (including beans, peas, and soybeans), shrimp and shellfish, fish, eggs, milk, wheat and wheat products, or corn and corn products.

The most likely culprits among the nuts are those that grow on trees: almonds, Brazil nuts, cashews, hazelnuts (filberts), hickory nuts, pecans, pine nuts (pignolis), pistachios, and especially walnuts. If you have had an allergic reaction to any one of these nuts, you are almost certainly allergic to the others as well.

Peanuts are legumes, not nuts, but they too are highly allergenic. If you are allergic to peanuts, you should avoid all peanut products, including peanut oil. You might also be allergic to other legumes, including beans, peas, soybeans, and soy products. Soy products are included in many packaged and processed foods—even ice cream—so read the labels carefully.

Shrimp and other shellfish can trigger severe allergic reactions, as can allergies to fish. If you are allergic to shrimp or prawns, also avoid abalone, clams, crayfish, lobster, octopus, oysters, scallops, snails (including land snails), and squid. If you are allergic to fish, avoid *all* fish in any form, including canned tuna and salmon.

Wheat, corn, and eggs are so widely used that they are difficult to avoid. Read the labels carefully on prepared and processed foods to avoid hidden uses. Fortunately, fewer people are allergic to these foods. (We'll discuss ways to avoid wheat in the section on celiac disease below.)

Other foods that can cause allergic reactions in some people include tomatoes, berries, and chocolate. Food allergies are very individual, however, so if you get hives, a rash, or some other allergic reaction after eating a specific food that is not discussed here, you are probably allergic to it and should avoid it in the future.

Some foods are almost certain to never cause an allergic reaction. If you are troubled by food allergies, you can safely eat apples, artichokes, carrots, lamb, lettuce, peaches, pears, and rice.

About 5 percent of asthmatics are sensitive to the salicylates found naturally in certain foods; people who do not have asthma but do have other allergies are also sometimes sensitive to salicylates. Foods that naturally contain salicylates include tea, root beer, corned beef, avocados, cucumbers, green peppers, olives, potatoes, tomatoes, and some fruits—particularly apples, berries (including strawberries), cherries, grapes, melons, peaches, and plums. The herbs willow bark, meadowsweet, cowslip and primrose (primula), chamomile, lady's mantle, yarrow, red clover flowers, and sweet violet and heartsease (viola) also contain salicylates and should be avoided. Since other, less common herbs may contain salicylates, people with this sensitivity should simply avoid all herbal remedies to be on the safe side.

Some asthmatics and sensitive individuals also react to sulfites, which are widely used as preservatives in foods and beverages. Sulfites are commonly used in restaurants and convenience foods to help preserve the freshness of shrimp, potatoes, dehydrated soups, and other foods. They are also found naturally in beer, wine, and dried fruits (especially apricots). Monosodium glutamate (MSG) is another widely used food preservative that is often added to processed foods and soups and is also found in soy sauce, meat tenderizers, and seasoned salts; it can trigger asthma attacks or allergic reactions in sensitive individuals. If you are sensitive to sulfites or MSG, be very careful to avoid these ingredients. Many but not all restaurants have responded to customer complaints and have stopped using sulfites and MSG, but these substances are still widely used in packaged and convenience foods. Your best defense is to read the labels carefully.

Although a migraine headache is not, strictly speaking, an allergy, some foods—especially those that naturally contain substances called amines—can trigger a migraine in susceptible people. This is because amines affect the diameter of blood vessels; if blood vessels open up (dilate) too widely, a migraine headache can ensue.

Amines of various sorts are found in many foods. Tyramine, for example, is found in aged cheeses, herring, organ meats, many nuts and seeds, peanuts, sauerkraut, and alcohol; octopamine is found in citrus fruits, and phenylethylamine is found in chocolate. Other foods that contain amines include most beans and legumes (pinto beans and lentils, for example) and fruits such as figs, dates, raisins, passion fruit, pineapple, papayas, avocados, red plums, and bananas. Aged, pickled, preserved, fermented, cured, or cultured foods can also be migraine triggers. If you get migraines, try avoiding alcoholic beverages, including beer and wine; sausage meats such as salami and pepperoni; cultured dairy products, such as sour cream and buttermilk; breads and cakes containing yeast; olives; and pickles.

Nitrites and nitrates, chemicals that are often added to processed foods, can also trigger migraine headaches. Processed meats such as sausage, ham, bacon, luncheon meats, and hot dogs often contain nitrites and nitrates. Monosodium glutamate (MSG) can be a migraine trigger for some people. The caffeine in coffee, tea, or soft drinks may also be a factor in migraines. Most doctors recommend that migraine sufferers limit their caffeine intake to no more than two cups a day.

Self-help steps   Generally speaking, the symptoms of an allergic reaction to a food will appear suddenly and go away on their own within several hours. For example, hives (urticaria)—small, very itchy, red, swollen bumps on the skin—usually do arise very suddenly and go away just as fast, often within an hour or two. Sometimes, however, hives can last for twenty-four hours or more. Generally, hives are annoying and itchy but not really dangerous. If you get hives in your mouth or throat, however, get medical help at once. If you are wheezing or having difficulty breathing from any food allergy, get medical help at once.

Like hives, rashes from food allergies generally appear suddenly and go away within a few hours. A cold compress sometimes help relieve the itching of hives and rashes.

Drugs   Over-the-counter drugs such as simethicone can help relieve the uncomfortable symptoms of gas and bloating from a food allergy. Nonprescription creams containing 1 percent cortisone are helpful in relieving itching from hives or rashes. If the hives or rash persist, a nonprescription antihistamine such as pseudoephedrine hydrochloride (Sudafed or the generic equivalent) or diphenhydramine hydrochloride (Benadryl or the generic equivalent) may relieve the symptoms. If the hives or rash do not go away within twenty-four hours, call your doctor. If the hives or rash are in your mouth or throat, get medical help at once.

Do not attempt to treat wheeziness or shortness of breath with over-the-counter drugs. Call your doctor.

If you are extremely sensitive to a particular food, your doctor may advise you to carry prescription antihistamines or even an injectable emergency dose of epinephrine to counter anaphylactic shock.

Alternative Treatments

Herbal therapy Although herbs such as devil's claw, goldenseal, burdock root, and dandelion are sometimes suggested to treat food allergies, herbal treatments are unlikely to be helpful. In fact, some could be harmful. People with food allergies tend to also have respiratory allergies to pollens such as ragweed. Goldenseal, a close relative of ragweed, could actually induce an allergic reaction in a sensitive individual.

Vitamin and mineral supplements In general, people with food allergies should select hypoallergenic vitamin and mineral supplements. These products are made without fillers containing potential allergens such as corn starch.

People with food allergies are often helped somewhat by taking supplements of the antioxidants vitamin C, vitamin E, and mixed carotenes (the building blocks of vitamin A). The reason is that antioxidant vitamins "mop up" the free radicals—the destructive byproducts of the inflammatory response created by the allergic reaction—before they can damage delicate cell membranes. We recommend 600 IU daily of vitamin E, 1,000 milligrams daily of vitamin C, and 10,000 IU of mixed carotenes. The minerals selenium and zinc are also helpful for improving antioxidant levels. We suggest taking 15 to 30 milligrams of zinc and 250 micrograms of selenium daily. Do not exceed the selenium dosage; any more can be toxic.

Other supplements　　Your body naturally produces the antioxidant enzyme glutathione to fight free radicals caused by normal metabolism and allergic reactions. Supplements of the amino acid cysteine, the major building block of glutathione, and of the other cofactors such as selenium that your body needs to produce this essential antioxidant can help your body soak up all those free radicals. We recommend taking three capsules daily of GSH 250 Master Glutathione Formula from Douglas Labs for two days after you have had an allergic reaction to a food.

Homeopathy　　The homeopathic remedy urtica, made from the stinging nettle plant, is used to relieve the symptoms of allergic hives. The usual dosage is one 6c pill or six drops of 6c liquid under the tongue every hour until the hives go away.

Combined Treatments

Diet and supplements　　Avoiding known allergens is the best approach to food allergies. If an allergic reaction does occur, the symptoms, though uncomfortable, will usually pass on their own within a few hours. To help your body recover from the reaction, take supplements of antioxidant vitamins, glutathione, and the cofactors selenium and zinc.

LACTOSE INTOLERANCE

People with lactose intolerance naturally produce very little of the digestive enzyme lactase. This means that they can't digest significant amounts of lactose, the predominant sugar in milk and many milk products. If you can't produce enough lactase to digest the dairy products you consume, the undigested lactose travels to the large intestine, where bacteria cause it to ferment. The end result is gas, bloating, diarrhea, cramps, and sometimes nausea. The symptoms usually begin about thirty minutes to two hours after eating or drinking foods that contain lactose.

Lactose intolerance is quite common—in fact, the majority of the world's population is lactase deficient. In America, some 30 to 50 million people are affected. Certain ethnic and racial populations are more widely affected than others. As many as 75 percent of all African-Americans and Native Americans and 90 percent of Asian Americans are lactose intolerant; many people of Mediterranean descent are also lactose intolerant. The condition is least common among persons of northern European descent. Lactose intolerance is not the same as an allergy to cow's milk—if you suspect a milk allergy in your child, see your pediatrician.

For most people, lactose intolerance is a condition that develops gradually. After you've reached the age of about three, your body naturally begins to produce less lactase, but the symptoms of lactose intolerance don't usually begin to show up until you are in your late teens or early twenties. Often, however, the symptoms develop gradually in older people as their bodies stop producing lactase. Many people never associate their symptoms with milk or dairy products in their diet. For this reason, health care providers usually check for lactose intolerance before looking for any other food intolerances or whenever a patient starts having digestive difficulties. People with irritable bowel syndrome, for example, often are also lactose intolerant and improve greatly when they remove milk and dairy products from their diet.

Diagnosing lactose intolerance is generally quite straightforward. The simplest approach is to drink a glass of milk and note if gas, cramps, diarrhea, and other symptoms follow soon after. For a more accurate picture that also provides the degree of intolerance, your health care provider may suggest a breath test. This is a noninvasive procedure that is quite accurate; it can be done at home or in your health care provider's office. The patient eats a low-fiber diet for twenty-four hours before the test, then eats a light dinner of rice and some protein such as chicken or tofu the night before. After that, no food and only water are taken for twelve hours before the test.

The breath test itself is very easy. The patient collects a breath sample in a special tube, then ingests a premeasured amount of lactose. Three more breath samples are then collected hourly. The samples are sent to a laboratory for analysis of their hydrogen and methane content plotted over time. An increase in exhaled hydrogen and methane indicates lactose intolerance; the amount of the increase indicates the severity of the problem.

Traditional Treatments

Diet Avoiding lactose is the best way to avoid the unpleasant symptoms of lactose intolerance. In general, any form of milk—whole, skim, low fat, cream, half-and-half, powdered, condensed, evaporated—should be avoided or used only in moderation. Butter, margarine, ice cream, and soft cheeses such as ricotta, cottage cheese, sour cream, farmer cheese, and the like often cause problems. Semisoft or hard cheeses such as Swiss or cheddar can usually be eaten in small amounts. Some of the lactose is predigested in fermented milk products such as yogurt, but only if live cultures are used—yogurt without live cultures will be just as bad as milk.

People vary in their degree of intolerance. Some may find that they can tolerate a small glass of milk but not a large one; others can eat ice cream but not drink milk. Often lactose-intolerant people can eat small amounts of dairy foods after a meal without difficulty. A small dish of ice cream for dessert after a large dinner, for example, may not cause any symptoms, while the same amount of ice cream as a mid-afternoon snack would quickly cause discomfort. Most people can determine their optimal level of tolerance to milk and dairy products through cautious trial and error.

If you are lactose intolerant, you can turn elsewhere for the important calcium, protein, B vitamins, and other benefits of milk. One way is using lactose-reduced milk, which is sold in most supermarkets under the brand name Lactaid. This milk has had the enzyme lactase added to it. The enzyme splits the lactose into two simpler sugars, glucose and galactose, so Lactaid tastes sweeter than regular milk. Only about 70 percent of the lactose is affected, however, so if you are severely lactose intolerant you may still get symptoms. An alternative to Lactaid is adding lactase to milk yourself. Lactase drops are easily available over-the-counter at drugstores. Add the drops to your regular milk according to the package directions; use more if you are very intolerant. The milk needs to stay in the refrigerator for twenty-four hours before it is used, but after that it can be drunk or used in any recipe.

Acidophilus milk, which is regular milk that has had live acidophilus bacteria added to it, can be helpful in mild cases. These bacteria naturally produce lactase, which helps you digest it. Unfortunately, heating the milk kills the bacteria, so acidophilus milk can't be used in cooking or be added to anything hot.

Cultured buttermilk has slightly less lactose than an equivalent amount of regular milk. All forms of milk—regular, low fat, 1 percent, 2 percent, and skim—contain about the same amount of lactose; goat's milk contains as much lactose as cow's milk. Soy milk, of course, has no lactose.

People who are lactose intolerant need to watch out for the hidden lactose that is often added to prepared foods. Bread and other baked goods, milk chocolate, processed breakfast cereals, instant potatoes, soups, breakfast drinks, powdered coffee creamer, whipped toppings, margarine, salad dressings, and prepared mixes for pancakes, biscuits, and cookies often contain lactose. Lactose is even found in hot dogs and luncheon meats—read the labels carefully. When reading the list of ingredients, look for the words milk, lactose, whey, casein, caseinate, sodium caseinate, curds, milk byproducts, dry milk solids, and nonfat dry milk powder. If any of these appear on the label, the product contains lactose.

Lactose is also used as the base for more than 20 percent of prescription drugs and about 6 percent of over-the-counter drugs. These products will be a problem only if you are severely lactose intolerant, however. If you are concerned, discuss the lactose content of the drug with your doctor or pharmacist.

If you can't drink milk or eat dairy products, you may have trouble getting enough calcium in your diet. The recommended dietary allowance of calcium for an adult male is 800 milligrams a day. To help prevent osteoporosis later in life, premenopausal women should get 1,000 milligrams per day—roughly the calcium in a quart of milk. Women who are menopausal should get 1,500 milligrams. To get this much calcium without milk, try eating other dairy products such as live-culture yogurt and semisoft cheese in quantities you can tolerate. Foods that are high in calcium but contain no lactose include broccoli, bok choy, kale, collard greens, turnip greens, salmon, sardines, tofu, and molasses. In addition, we recommend calcium supplements, especially those that contain elemental calcium carbonate, since other forms of calcium will not be absorbed well by your body.

Drugs Nonprescription lactase tablets or drops can be purchased at any drugstore (popular brands include Lactaid and Dairy Ease). When you eat something that contains lactose, try chewing or swallowing one or two tablets first. You may have to experiment a bit to find the right dose, but the tablets do help, at least somewhat, by providing the missing enzyme. As discussed above, lactase drops can be added to milk in advance.

Alternative Treatments

The alternative treatments for lactose intolerance are the same as the traditional treatments.

FOOD INTOLERANCES

Food intolerances are nonallergic but very real reactions to foods. The onset of the symptoms is often delayed by twenty-four or even forty-eight hours, and the reactions do not usually involve the immune system. Food intolerance symptoms are less specific and more widespread than those of food allergies. As we discussed above, the symptoms of food intolerance are easily confused with lactose intolerance, particularly because many foods contain hidden lactose. (We'll discuss celiac disease, a fairly rare condition that affects the ability to digest wheat and other foods, at the end of this chapter.) Gastrointestinal ailments such as gastroesophageal reflux disease (GERD), irritable bowel syndrome, and gallbladder problems can also mimic food intolerances. Finally, some health care practitioners believe that many if not all cases of food intolerance are caused not by a particular food but by absorption problems in the small intestine, which are themselves caused by leaky gut syndrome or by dysbiosis. Because small intestine problems can account for so many cases of food intolerance, information in both this section and in chapter 6, on problems of the small intestine, is pertinent.

The first step in diagnosing food intolerance is to realize that it may be responsible for your poor health. As you can see from table 5.1, the symptoms of food intolerance include mental states and physical problems that may seem far removed from the foods you eat. The symptoms may also come and go and change from day to day. This is a normal effect of a reaction to a food you don't eat every day, but many traditional physicians tend to dismiss changeable or vague symptoms as imaginary or psychological, not medical. If, however, you can realistically find no other reason for the array of symptoms you feel, you should seriously consider food intolerances as their cause.

5.1

FOOD INTOLERANCE SYMPTOMS

General Symptoms
- overall feeling of ill health
- constant exhaustion
- "flu-like" symptoms
- feeling worse after eating, better after fasting
- sudden weight loss or gain
- fluid retention or swelling, especially around the ankles

Eyes
- burning or gritty feeling
- dark or puffy circles under the eyes
- redness or bloodshot eyes
- watering

Gastrointestinal
- appetite loss/gain
- bloating
- constipation
- cramps
- diarrhea
- gas
- heartburn
- indigestion

Lungs
- asthma
- dry cough
- wheeziness

Mouth and Throat
- bad or metallic taste in mouth
- cold sores
- difficulty swallowing

Table 5.1 (cont)

dry mouth	mood swings
hoarseness	poor concentration
increased salivation	poor memory
mouth ulcers	restlessness
sore throat	*Sinuses, Nose, Ears*
Muscles and Joints	earaches
muscle cramps	hearing loss
muscle or joint stiffness	itching
swollen joints	nasal congestion or stuffi-
muscle weakness	ness
Nervous System/Mental State	postnasal drip
anxiety	runny nose
confusion	sinus pain or headaches
depression	sneezing
dizziness	tinnitus (ringing in ears)
fatigue	*Skin*
"fogginess" or inability to	acne
think clearly	eczema
headaches	hives
insomnia	itching
irritability	rashes

Source: Dr. Alan Pressman, Gramercy Health Associates

Not surprisingly, the many possible alternative causes of food intolerances can make specific intolerances hard to identify. You don't need a battery of expensive laboratory tests to determine your food intolerances. An elimination diet that removes suspect foods and gradually adds them back until the culprits turn up is relatively easy to follow on your own, with the advice of your health care provider.

Begin by making a list of all the foods you normally

eat more than three or four times a week. Be sure to include everything — even no-calorie breath mints. The reason for making the list is that your food intolerances may be the result of prolonged exposure to foods you eat often. Also list the foods you find yourself craving, such as ice cream, milk, chocolate, or salty snacks, as well as foods you intuitively know make you feel worse. The next step is by far the hardest—eliminate all the foods on your list from your diet for two to three entire weeks. That doesn't mean you have to starve yourself, although many patients do lose a few unwanted pounds as an unexpected bonus. Work with your health care provider to find nutritionally equivalent foods for those you have eliminated. Since almost everyone can eat apples, artichokes, carrots, lamb, lettuce, peaches, pears, and rice without reacting, these foods can be the starting points for diet substitutions. In severe cases, you may have to eat nothing but these foods for the first fourteen days. Be sure to drink six to eight glasses of pure water every day.

As you go through the elimination part of the program, keep a record of how you feel. During the first few days of your elimination diet, your symptoms may actually get a little worse as your body adjusts, but by the end of the first week they should be improved. After two to three weeks without your most frequently eaten foods, your symptoms should be markedly better. If they're not, look carefully at your diet. Are you really sticking to it? Are you inadvertently eating foods that contain items on your elimination list? You may have another underlying condition that is causing the problem. Discuss the situation with your health care provider.

The next step in your program is to reintroduce the

foods you have eliminated to find out which ones cause symptoms. It's especially important to keep your food journal on a regular basis during the reintroduction period.

Start by looking at the foods on your elimination list. As you know from the food allergies section above, foods such as nuts, eggs, and seafood are likely to be allergenic. Skip over those foods for now and select some other food to reintroduce.

At breakfast on day one of the reintroduction, eat a large helping of the food along with your regular elimination-diet foods. Make a note of any sensations or symptoms you experience soon after eating the food. It's possible that the food will make you feel unusually good or even high. If you have a reaction soon after eating the food, you are intolerant of it. If you have no reaction, eat another helping at lunch. If there is still no reaction, make a note of it in your journal and drop the food for now.

For the next three days, observe yourself for any delayed reactions to the food you ate on day one. Often food intolerances produce symptoms only twenty-four to forty-eight hours after exposure.

On the next four-day cycle, reintroduce a different food and again note your responses. Continue for as long as necessary to reintroduce the foods you most commonly eat. Continue to keep your food journal during this period. By looking at your journal after several weeks of reintroductions, you will easily see which foods are safe, which produce immediate reactions, and which produce delayed reactions.

Once you've determined your food intolerances, you can then discover the treatments that work best for you.

Traditional Treatments

Diet If you know a particular food causes an undesirable response, avoid it. If you have multiple food intolerances or allergies, however, your diet could become very restricted, to the point of not providing sufficient nutrients and variety. Many of our patients benefit from a low-fat diet rich in fresh fruits, vegetables, and whole grains and low in meats, dairy products, and processed foods; they also often find that a rotation diet, which provides many different safe foods and limits their reactive foods to only once every few days or less, lets them eat interesting and nutritious foods without causing symptoms. The rotary diversified diet, as this is often called, is a medically well-accepted program that helps reduce and relieve food intolerances. The diet takes some getting used to, mostly because it calls for different foods every day. If you are accustomed to having bread with every meal or oatmeal for breakfast every day, for example, the change might be hard at first. This diet works on the principle of rotating foods that are safe for you on a five- or six-day cycle. So, for example, if you eat spinach on a Monday, you cannot have it again until Saturday or Sunday. This diet helps to keep food sensitivities from acting up. Although this diet is actually fairly straightforward and easy to follow, it requires more explanation than we have room for here. You'll probably feel so much better, that you'll get used to it quickly. Your health care practitioner can help you get started with basic menus.

The basic principles of the rotation diets are outlined in the works of the pioneering physician Theron Randolph—for instance, *An Alternative Approach to Allergies* (New York: HarperCollins, 1990). The practical aspects of the rotation diet are presented in *Dr. Mandell's Five Day Allergy Relief System*, by Marshall Mandell, M.D., and Lynn Walter Scanlon (New York: T.Y. Crowell, 1979).

Alternative Treatments

Several alternative methods of determining food intolerances are sometimes recommended by alternative practitioners. These include cytotoxic testing, sublingual provocation-neutralization tests, pulse testing, electronic screening, and applied kinesiology or biokinesiology testing. Unfortunately, none of these methods is reliable enough to replace the elimination diet discussed above. Most alternative practitioners would agree that the rotary diversified diet is the most effective way to deal with food intolerances.

Vitamin and mineral supplements Although the elimination and rotary diversified diets are nutritionally complete, we recommend taking a good daily vitamin and mineral supplement. Be sure to select a product that is hypoallergenic and contains no wheat, cornstarch, lactose, or other fillers. Women on the rotary diversified diet may not be getting enough calcium to help prevent osteoporosis later in life. They should keep in mind that the recommended daily amount of calcium for premenopausal women is 1,000 milligrams; for women who are menopausal, the daily requirement is 1,500 milligrams. We recommend calcium supplements to all our women patients, but especially to those with restricted diets.

Other supplements The amino acid glutamine and gamma oryzanol (rice bran oil) are helpful for nourishing and healing the intestines while you are on the elimination diet. The recommended daily dose is 5,000 milligrams of glutamine, with the doses spread out evenly over the day. A capsule of rice bran oil with each meal may also help.

Combined Treatments

Diet and supplements Use the elimination diet to determine your food intolerances and the rotary diversified diet to keep them under control. Vitamin and mineral supplements, along with glutamine and rice bran oil, help maintain your nutritional status and heal your digestive system.

CELIAC DISEASE

Celiac disease is an allergy to gluten, a protein found in wheat, oats, barley, and rye. Also known as gluten-sensitive enteropathy, sprue, celiac sprue, or nontropical sprue, celiac disease is fairly uncommon, affecting no more than six Americans in every 10,000. The symptoms, including irritability, poor absorption of nutrients, weight loss, gas, abdominal bloating, greasy stools, and diarrhea, often begin in infancy or early childhood when cereal foods are introduced to the diet. More rarely, celiac disease begins in young adults between the ages of twenty and thirty. If you have celiac disease, you will have it for life, although it may be quiescent during the adolescent years.

Traditional Treatments

Diet   There is no cure for celiac disease. The only treatment is to avoid gluten in any form. Unfortunately, this is difficult to do, given the usual wheat-based diet of Western society. Gluten is found in any food that contains wheat, oats, barley, or rye, including bread, pasta, cereal, baked goods, and beer. Hidden gluten is found in many processed or prepared foods, including salad dressings, gravies, soups, and ice cream. Even though corn is acceptable, for example, commercial cornbread mixes contain more wheat than corn. Celiacs must read food labels very carefully to avoid hidden problem foods. Check the ingredients list for the words malt, malt flavoring, malt coloring, bran, farina, semolina, hydrolyzed vegetable protein (HVP), hydrolyzed plant protein (HPP), modified food starch, vegetable gum, monosodium glutamate (MSG), or grain (white) vinegar. These additives all contain gluten.

Most patients who have just been diagnosed with celiac disease have already suffered damage to the lining of their small intestine and can't absorb nutrients from their food properly. Because of this and because celiac disease is not always diagnosed quickly, these patients are often underweight and badly nourished. Fortunately, once gluten has been eliminated from the diet, intestinal healing begins. During this time, the small intestine also can't produce the digestive enzyme lactase, so celiac patients may also be temporarily lactose intolerant as well. Celiac patients may have to avoid lactose and fatty foods, but they can usually add these back to the diet within six months.

Constant, lifelong vigilance is the only way celiacs

can avoid eating gluten and causing a flare-up of symptoms. Be very cautious of new foods. Even a trace of gluten will cause symptoms to appear within twenty-four hours—and possibly as soon as within twenty minutes. The reaction—with all its unpleasant, debilitating symptoms—could last anywhere from a day or so up to ten days.

Many of the less common grains touted as health foods that are safe for people with allergies can still cause severe problems for celiacs. Avoid amaranth, buckwheat, bulgur, kamut, millet, quinoa, semolina, spelt, teff, and triticale. Some celiacs also react to soy products.

Despite the restrictions, many tasty recipes using rice, corn, artichoke flour, nuts, potatoes, and other safe foods have been developed for celiacs, and it is possible with some extra care to eat an interesting and nutritious diet. Dietary fiber usually helps the condition, so celiacs should eat lots of fresh fruits and vegetables, especially beans, nuts, berries, and seeds. Even so, the celiac diet can lead to vitamin and mineral deficiencies. Your doctor will probably prescribe a multivitamin with minerals and also an additional B vitamin supplement. While your small intestine is healing, you may need regular injections of B vitamins. Your doctor may also recommend free-form amino acid protein supplements during this time.

Once your physician has diagnosed celiac disease, ask for a referral to a nutritionist who can help you learn to detect hidden gluten, prepare safe foods for yourself, and select safe foods when eating out. You may also want to meet with other celiacs for mutual help. For information about a celiac support group near you, contact:

Celiac Sprue Association
Box 31700
Omaha, NE 68131-0700
(402) 558-0600

or

Gluten Intolerance Group of North America
Box 23053
Seattle, WA 98102-0353
(206) 325-6980

Alternative Treatments

The alternative treatments for celiac disease are the same as the traditional treatments.

CHAPTER 6

Problems of the Small Intestine

After several hours in your stomach, the food you have eaten has been churned up into a soupy, very acidic mixture called chyme. As part of normal digestion, the pyloric valve at the lower end of your stomach opens and empties the chyme into the small intestine. Some fifteen to twenty feet long but only about an inch and a half wide, your small intestine is where the real work of nourishing your body takes place.

Peristalsis, the normal, involuntary movement of the intestines, carries the chyme from the stomach into the duodenum, a portion of the small intestine that is about twelve to eighteen inches long. Here the hydrochloric acid from your stomach is rapidly neutralized by bicarbonate produced by your pancreas. Additional digestive enzymes from your pancreas, gallbladder, and the small intestine itself are added now as peristalsis slowly propels the chyme onward through the small intestine into the jejunum, the ten-foot-long middle section of your small intestine. From the jejunum, the chyme moves on to the final portion of the small intestine, the twelve-foot-long ileum.

Digestive enzymes break up the proteins into their individual amino acids, while carbohydrates are converted to simpler sugars, and fats are emulsified into tiny globules and then broken down into fatty acids and glycerol.

The nutrients are absorbed into your bloodstream by millions of tiny, fingerlike projections called villi that line the inside of your small intestine and vastly enlarge its total surface area (your small intestine has about the same surface area as a tennis court). The dense network of tiny blood vessels surrounding the villi carry the nutrients to your liver for further processing. The cells lining your small intestine are continually being replaced by new cells; the old lining is shed and eliminated along with other waste products.

Different nutrients are absorbed at different points along the small intestine. The fat-soluble vitamins A, D, and E are absorbed in the duodenum, along with vitamin C and some of the B vitamins. Minerals such as calcium and iron are absorbed at this point, as are fats and some sugars. In the jejunum, the water-soluble B vitamins (thiamine, pyridoxine, riboflavin, folic acid) are absorbed, along with proteins, amino acids, and sugars such as lactose and sucrose. Cholesterol, vitamin B_{12}, and bile salts from your gallbladder are absorbed in the ileum. By the time your food has passed all the way through your small intestine, only water, indigestible fiber, living and dead bacteria, and the debris shed normally from the intestinal lining should be left to enter your colon.

Clearly, problems in the small intestine will keep you from absorbing and assimilating food properly, which in turn will lead to uncomfortable symptoms, illness, and poor nutrition. Small-intestine problems can be caused by or mistaken for food allergies and intolerances (and vice versa). If you think you may have a small-intestine ailment, please be sure to read chapter 5 on food allergies. Crohn's disease, a problem that affects the ileum and often also the colon, will be discussed in chapter 9, on large intestine problems.

PANCREATIC INSUFFICIENCY

When the contents of your stomach enter your duodenum, the hydrochloric acid and pepsin of your digestive juices are neutralized by bicarbonate compounds produced by the exocrine portion of your pancreas. (The endocrine portion of your pancreas also, incidentally, produces insulin and other hormones for regulating your blood sugar.) The acidic chyme coming from your stomach also stimulates cells in the lining of your duodenum to secrete two hormones—secretin and cholecystokinin—that in turn stimulate the exocrine portion of the pancreas to release a number of digestive enzymes into the duodenum at this time. Proteins in food are broken down into their component amino acids by the enzymes trypsin and chymotrypsin, while starches are broken down by various amylase and saccharidase enzymes, and fats are broken down by lipase, yet another enzyme. Bile salts from your gallbladder enter the duodenum and help digest fats.

The digestive enzymes produced by the pancreas are essential to proper assimilation of food. Pancreatic insufficiency—the failure to produce adequate levels of digestive enzymes—can lead to malabsorption and other digestive difficulties. If your pancreas doesn't produce enough protease enzymes, for example, protein particles could enter your bloodstream and trigger an allergic response. If your pancreas doesn't produce enough of the complex fat-digesting enzymes, your body won't be able to absorb enough of the essential fatty acids it needs to make prostaglandins and other hormones.

The most common symptoms of pancreatic insufficiency include gas, bloating, heartburn, indigestion, diarrhea, and stools with undigested food in them. Food allergies and intolerances may also indicate pancreatic insufficiency.

Serious cases of pancreatic insufficiency leading to an inability to digest fats are rare, but many health care practitioners believe that low levels of chronic pancreatic insufficiency are fairly common and are at the root of many digestive problems. Because the acidity of the chyme triggers the production of the enzymes, people who produce too little stomach acid (hypochlorhydria) may suffer from pancreatic insufficiency due to lack of acid stimulation. (See chapter 2 on heartburn for more information about hypochlorhydria.)

To diagnose pancreatic insufficiency, your doctor will send your stool sample to a laboratory and have it checked for fecal fat. If your pancreas is functioning normally, most of the fat you eat will be absorbed in your small intestine and very little will be excreted in your stool. In most cases, a single stool sample is sufficient. In some cases, however, you may need to collect all your stool over a seventy-two-hour period.

A comprehensive digestive stool analysis (CDSA) is another way of determining if you have pancreatic insufficiency. This test looks at your stool sample for levels of the enzyme chymotrypsin, triglycerides, and the presence of undigested meat and vegetable fibers. Low levels of chymotrypsin, high levels of triglycerides (the major component in dietary fat), and the presence of undigested food all suggest reduced pancreatic output.

Traditional Treatments

Diet Pancreatic insufficiency can have several causes. One is a sudden, large change in diet. People who suddenly add a lot more fiber to their diet, for example, may suffer from excessive gas while their pancreas adapts to the change by producing more of some enzymes and less of others. To avoid this sort of digestive difficulty, make dietary changes gradually.

Many practitioners feel that a diet too low in fiber or too high in sugar can cause the pancreas to reduce its output of enzymes. If you have the symptoms of pancreatic insufficiency, slowly adding more fiber to your diet by eating plenty of fresh fruits and vegetables could help quite a bit. Cutting back on sugar could also help.

How much liquid a patient with pancreatic insufficiency should drink with meals is somewhat controversial among health care practitioners. Some believe that too much fluid dilutes the gastric juices in the stomach and the pancreatic enzymes in the duodenum. Others believe that inadequate fluids with meals may be a cause of the problem, since fluids also stimulate the production of gastric juices and digestive enzymes. In our experience, drinking one or two glasses of pure water with every meal usually helps our patients. If you feel that drinking with every meal is not helping or is making your symptoms worse, however, drink less or nothing with meals. However, you should then be sure to drink six to eight glasses of water a day in between meals instead.

Drugs Drugs that contain pancreatic enzymes derived from animal glands are called pancreatins. The most common prescription drug for pancreatic insufficiency is generically known as pancrelipase or lipancreatin. Brand names include Cotazym, Entolase, Festal, Ilozyme, Ku-Zyme, Viokase, and Zymase. The enteric-coated form of these drugs is usually prescribed to keep the enzymes from being denatured (destroyed) by digestive juices in the stomach before they reach the duodenum. Generally, if your doctor prescribes pancrelipase for you, he or she will also prescribe a low-fat, low-sugar diet. A drug known by the brand name Donnazyme is a more powerful treatment for pancreatic insufficiency. This drug contains pancreatin, pepsin, bile salts, and several other potent drugs, including atropine and phenobarbital. If your doctor prescribes Donnazyme, he or she will also prescribe a special diet and caution you about possible side effects and drug interactions.

Alternative Treatments

Herbal therapy   In traditional European herbal medicine, bitter-tasting herbs are believed to stimulate the flow of digestive juices, including those from the pancreas. The bitter herb usually recommended for pancreatic insufficiency is gentian root *(Gentiana lutea)*. The principal flavoring in angostura bitters, gentian is also generally recommended as an appetite stimulant. To make gentian tea, boil one teaspoon of powdered gentian root in half a cup of water for five minutes. Strain before drinking. Most herbalists recommend drinking gentian tea half an hour before mealtime; have no more than two cups daily.

In traditional Chinese medicine, ginseng tea is said to be an appetite stimulant that also improves the flow of digestive juices. Ginseng is usually taken as a tea made from the powdered root. To prepare ginseng tea, steep one to three teaspoons of ginseng in one cup boiling water for ten minutes, stirring occasionally. Stir before drinking. Ginseng tablets and capsules are available in various dosages. Herbalists generally suggest daily doses ranging from 500 milligrams to two grams. To help the symptoms of pancreatic insufficiency, try drinking a cup of the tea or taking a capsule after meals.

A South African plant called devil's claw *(Harpagophytum procumbens)* is sometimes recommended as a bitter along the lines of gentian root. Try taking one capsule after a meal.

Supplements Some practitioners recommend supplemental digestive enzymes for patients with mild symptoms of pancreatic insufficiency. Papain, the digestive enzyme found naturally in papaya, and bromelain, the digestive enzyme found naturally in pineapple, are helpful for digesting protein. Tablets and capsules containing papain and bromelain are available at health food stores. Take one or two at the start of each meal. Enzymes made from the fungus *Aspergillus oryzae* may also be helpful for improving stomach and pancreatic function. Take one or two capsules at the start of each meal.

Glandular-based supplements made from pig pancreases are available at health food stores. The strengths of these supplements are indicated by the standard United States Pharmacopoeia (USP) scale and usually range from 4x to 10x. The higher the number, the more potent the product is said to be. Health care practitioners usually suggest taking 8x or 10x preparations, since lower-potency products are often diluted with lactose or other fillers. The usual dosage is one to two capsules or tablets just before meals. Avoid raw glandular products. Animal diseases could be passed on to you.

Store all digestive enzyme products in the refrigerator to keep them from breaking down.

Juice therapy   A more enjoyable and also more caloric way of getting the natural digestive enzyme bromelain is drinking fresh, unsweetened pineapple juice. Try having an eight-ounce glass about fifteen minutes before each meal. Because pineapple juice is very high in natural sugars, don't drink it if you have diabetes, hypoglycemia, or any sort of blood sugar problem. Papain, the digestive enzyme found in papaya, is most abundant in the unripe fruit, which is hard and bitter. Fresh papaya juice made from ripe fruit will not have much papain in it, although it is delicious and an excellent source of vitamin C.

Relaxation techniques   If you are under a lot of stress or are very tense when you eat, your output of pancreatic enzymes will probably be reduced, with undesirable effects. Try to eat your meals in a calm, relaxed, unhurried atmosphere. Chew your food thoroughly.

Combined Treatments

Diet and supplements   A high-fiber, low-fat, low-sugar diet can help normalize the production of your pancreatic enzymes. Drink one to two glasses of pure water with each meal; if this does not help, reduce the amount of fluid you drink with meals. If your meal includes animal protein or dairy products, try taking bromelain or papain tablets with the meal to aid in digestion. If you have normal blood sugar and don't need to worry about the

extra calories, try a glass of fresh pineapple juice instead
of the bromelain tablets.

DYSBIOSIS

As a rule, your small intestine is a relatively sterile environment. The high acid levels of your stomach tend to kill
most bacteria and other pathogens that we eat, and the
constant movement of the chyme through your small intestine keeps bacteria from growing very well. Even so,
your small intestine contains billions of bacteria that not
only aid in digestion but actually manufacture some of
the vitamins you need. In fact, without all those friendly
bacteria your digestion would be seriously impaired.
(As we'll discuss in chapter 9, your large intestine is
crammed with *trillions* of bacteria.) Along with literally
hundreds of different kinds of friendly bacteria, however,
your intestines also host some not-so-friendly or down-
right hostile bacteria. The delicate balance of good and
bad bacteria can be disrupted by illness, injury, drugs,
insufficient stomach acid (hypochlorhydria), pancreatic
insufficiency, parasites, or poor diet—alone or in combination. In that case, the altered intestinal environment can
favor the growth of one type of bacteria over all the others; it can also let yeastlike organisms such as *Candida
albicans* crowd out other organisms. The result is dysbiosis—a condition where undesirable gut organisms badly
outnumber friendly organisms.

When the undesirable bacteria multiply in your small
intestine, the enzymes they produce can interfere with the
digestive enzymes that your body produces. The bad bacteria can also prevent nutrients from being absorbed
through the villi. Eventually, dysbiosis can damage the

villi and the delicate mucus membrane that covers them, leading to leaky gut syndrome.

As you can see from chart 6.1, many persistent digestive problems can be traced back to dysbiosis. If you frequently have gas, bloating, diarrhea, or abdominal cramps within one or two hours of eating, dysbiosis may be the cause. If you frequently get vaginal yeast infections or have respiratory allergies, eczema, or psoriasis, intestinal dysbiosis could be the real culprit. You could also experience mental and emotional symptoms such as depression and difficulty concentrating. You might have deficiencies of vitamin K and vitamin B_{12}. In the long run, dysbiosis can lead to weight loss, poor nutrition, chronic fatigue, anemia, and increased susceptibility to infection. Years of poor calcium absorption could lead to osteoporosis.

Many health care practitioners are starting to realize that dysbiosis is fairly common. Compare your symptoms to those in chart 6.1; if you have had more than two of the symptoms over the past six weeks, bacterial overgrowth could be the problem and you should consult your doctor.

Some simple, noninvasive lab tests can verify bacterial overgrowth. A comprehensive digestive stool analysis (CDSA) can reveal evidence of hypochlorhydria (a common underlying cause of dysbiosis) or of poor digestion or malabsorption. These conditions strongly hint at dysbiosis, but other problems could be the cause. Lactose intolerance, for example, must be ruled out.

For a more certain diagnosis, many health care practitioners recommend a breath test for bacterial overgrowth of the small intestine. This test is easy to do and is considered to be quite accurate; your health care practitioner

Chart 6.1

BACTERIAL OVERGROWTH SYMPTOMS

Within one to two hours of eating:
  gas
  bloating (especially in lower abdomen)
  diarrhea
  cramps
Over a period of several days or more:
  weight loss
  fatigue
  depression
  difficulty concentrating

anemia
increased susceptibility to infection
PMS
vaginal yeast infection
respiratory allergy symptoms (sinusitis, rhinitis, bronchitis)
skin allergy symptoms (eczema, dermatitis)

Source: Great Smokies Diagnostic Laboratory, 1996.

---

can provide you with a test kit to do the test at home. Start by eating a simple protein and rice meal the night before; avoid high-fiber foods for twenty-four hours before the test. After your evening meal, do not eat anything else or drink anything but pure water. The next morning, you will breathe into a special tube to collect a fasting breath sample. The next step is to drink a premixed solution containing lactulose, a sugar that produces hydrogen or methane gas when it is digested by bacteria in your intestines but is not actually absorbed into your body. After you drink the lactulose, collect a sample of your breath in the special tubes provided by the test kit every fifteen minutes for the next two hours. Package the breath samples according to the kit directions and send them off to the lab. Your health care practitioner will receive the results soon after.

If you exhale extra hydrogen or methane gas, it is an indication that bacteria in your small intestine are digesting the lactulose, which in turn indicates dysbiosis. If you don't have a bacterial overgrowth, the lactulose will pass undigested through your small intestine and you won't exhale any extra gases. One drawback of this test is that some very sensitive patients may have cramping or minor diarrhea from the lactulose.

An alternative to using lactulose for the breath test is using glucose. The procedure and results are very similar, but this test is not appropriate for anyone with diabetes, hypoglycemia, or any sort of blood sugar disorder.

Even with proper and consistent treatment, dysbiosis often takes several weeks or even months to clear up. It's important to continue with your treatment program even if you don't notice an immediate improvement. If you keep with it, you'll probably start to notice a slight improvement after the first couple of weeks and a more significant improvement by six weeks.

Traditional Treatments

Diet   A low-starch or low-sugar diet may help restore a favorable balance of bacteria. If your overgrowth is in the jejunum (the first part of the small intestine) try cutting back on sugar, especially refined sugar, in your diet. If the overgrowth is in the ileum (the lower portion of your small intestine) cutting back on starchy foods may help more. In either case, eating more insoluble fiber may help quite a bit by making your food move through your small intestine more quickly. In mild cases that do not involve *Candida albicans* (yeast), adding fermented dairy products such as unflavored live-culture yogurt can help by restoring some favorable bacteria to your small intestine. Most supermarket yogurts do not contain live cultures, so you'll probably have to purchase live-culture yogurt at a health food store. Try having several ounces just before each meal.

Drugs Ironically, the overuse of prescription antibiotic drugs is one of the causes of dysbiosis. Drugs such as penicillin kill off all aerobic bacteria, both good and bad, and can open the way for undesirable anaerobic bacteria and *Candida albicans* to colonize the small intestine. In years past, another antibiotic, tetracycline, was sometimes prescribed for intestinal overgrowth. Because many microbes have become resistant to this drug, however, more than half of all patients aren't helped by it any longer. Broad-spectrum antibiotics such as amoxicillin or metronidazole (Flagyl) are more useful.

Alternative Treatments
Beneficial bacteria supplements Many patients benefit from a two-step approach that restores beneficial bacteria to the small intestine and also provides nutrients that help them become reestablished. The beneficial bacteria multiply with the help of the nutrients and crowd out the bad bacteria and yeast.

Supplements of high-quality acidophilus, bulgaricus, bifidobacteria, or lactobacillus in powder form help restore beneficial bacteria. Many different beneficial bacteria supplements are available. To select a good product, look for those that contain only one type of bacteria, preferably the DDS-1 acidophilus strain or the Malyoth bifidobacteria strain. The product should be cultured in a milk-based medium and then ultrafiltered, not centrifuged. Finally, the product should be certified to contain at least one billion (yes, *billion*) active bacteria per gram. Purchase the supplement only if you know that it has been kept refrigerated and does not contain the bacteria *Lactobacillus casei* or *Streptococcus faecium*.

To get the maximum benefit from friendly bacteria supplements, combine acidophilus and bifidobacteria supplements. The usual daily dosage for a mild bacterial overgrowth problem is one gram (about half a level teaspoon) of acidophilus with 250 milligrams (about an eighth of a teaspoon) of bifidobacteria. Mix the powders in three ounces of pure, chlorine-free cold water, and drink it on an empty stomach about ten to fifteen minutes before eating. Taking the bacteria on an empty stomach seems to help them survive the powerful acids of the stomach and the first part of the small intestine, and arrive safely in the ileum (lower portion of the small intestine). If you prefer, take the bacteria in capsules with a full glass of pure water.

If you have a serious bacterial overgrowth or if your overgrowth is affecting your liver function, you may need to take between five and ten grams of acidophilus and up to six grams of bifidobacteria daily, spread out between meals during the day. In addition, you may wish to add supplements of *Lactobacillus bulgarica*. These bacteria are most effective when three to six grams are taken with meals.

Once bacteria arrive in the proper part of your small intestine, they need some nutritional help to regain their foothold. Most practitioners recommend taking fructooligosaccharides (FOS) along with beneficial bacteria supplements. Supplements of FOS fuel the growth of beneficial bacteria in the gut. Because they are not broken down and digested by your body, they are completely available only to the bacteria. Low levels of FOS are found naturally in some foods such as honey and garlic; artichoke flour contains higher levels of FOS. To get the real benefits of FOS, however, the higher concentrations of 95 percent pure powder or syrup are most helpful. FOS products are mildly sweet and can be used as a sweetener in beverages or on food, although they don't work very well as a sugar substitute in cooking. Alternatively, you can swallow them as tablets. Start with one gram (about a quarter teaspoon) a day and gradually increase the dose to three or four grams daily. Large amounts of FOS can cause mild diarrhea in some people. If this occurs, reduce your daily dose until you return to normal.

When you start to take beneficial bacteria for dysbiosis, you may have a temporary worsening of symptoms, including gas and diarrhea, as the bad bacteria die off suddenly and release toxins. Although this is perfectly normal, you can avoid the discomfort by starting with small doses and gradually increasing them. Cut back on the dosage if your symptoms become too unpleasant.

Other supplements   The amino acid glutamine is vital for nourishing the cells that line your small intestine, but bacterial overgrowth can keep glutamine from reaching the lining. This can slow your recovery from dysbiosis and, as we'll discuss below, could cause leaky gut syndrome. Glutamine tablets are available at health food stores; take one 500-milligram glutamine capsule four times a day until your dysbiosis has cleared up.

Juice therapy   Cabbage juice is naturally very high in glutamine. If you prefer, try substituting eight ounces of fresh cabbage juice for one or two of the glutamine capsules.

Combined Treatments

Diet and beneficial bacteria supplements   Changing your diet and adding beneficial bacteria supplements is usually very helpful for clearing up dysbiosis. It is vital to reduce the amounts of sugars and starches you eat and to increase the amounts of insoluble fiber in your diet. At the same time, begin taking beneficial bacteria supplements and FOS. Start with small doses and gradually increase them. Continue for at least six weeks or until your symptoms are gone.

LEAKY GUT SYNDROME

Your small intestine absorbs nutrients through the delicate mucous membrane covering the villi. That same lining is an important barrier that excludes toxins, bacteria, large molecules, and particles of undigested food. Ordinarily, your intestinal lining is very "tight." Only small molecules of digested nutrients such as amino acids and peptides (short chains of amino acids) should be able to pass through the membrane and be absorbed into your bloodstream. But if your small intestine has been damaged by poor diet, illness, high stress levels, or certain drugs, or if you have food allergies, you could develop increased intestinal permeability—more familiarly known as leaky gut syndrome. The damage makes your small intestine become more permeable, which could allow toxins, microbes, and larger molecules of incompletely digested food to enter your bloodstream. Your body often reacts to the large molecules (also called endotoxins, which means toxins from within) as if they were allergy triggers. If you have leaky gut syndrome, you might develop symptoms of allergic reaction, including inflammation, rashes, diarrhea, joint pain, or even asthma. In more serious cases, you could develop an illness such as Crohn's disease, rheumatoid arthritis, psoriasis, or some other chronic, debilitating condition.

Increased intestinal permeability can cause chronic irritation of the gut lining. This, in turn, can lead to impaired digestion and malabsorption of critical nutrients, leading to nutritional deficiencies. Because toxic substances can pass into your bloodstream from the "leaks" in your small intestine, your liver—the organ responsible for removing toxins—comes under stress.

Some illnesses or the treatments for them can actually cause leaky gut syndrome. Examples include inflammatory bowel disease, HIV infection or AIDS, pancreatic insufficiency, celiac disease, food allergies, and parasite infestation. If you have been treated with nonsteroidal anti-inflammatory drugs (NSAIDs), steroid drugs, or antibiotics, or if you have been frequently exposed to environmental toxins or alcohol, you could have leaky gut syndrome.

Holistic health practitioners are starting to realize that leaky gut syndrome is at the root of a lot of chronic poor health and that it is fairly common. If you think that a leaky gut is causing some of your health problems, look at the symptoms listed in chart 6.2. If you have had more than two of the symptoms over the past four to six weeks, leaky gut syndrome could be the cause.

A simple, noninvasive test you can obtain from your

Chart 6.2

LEAKY GUT SYNDROME SYMPTOMS

Physical Symptoms	Mental/Emotional Symptoms
bloating	depression
gas	mood swings
cramps	poor memory
diarrhea	anxiety or nervousness
constipation	fatigue
fatigue	confused or "fuzzy"
food allergies	thinking
skin rashes	
headaches	
joint pain	
frequent colds and minor	
illnesses	

Source: Dr. Alan Pressman

health care provider and do at home can provide evidence of intestinal permeability and tell you how severe the problem is. The first step is to collect a urine specimen in the container provided with the kit at any convenient time the day before you do the test. That night, have a simple evening meal and do not eat or drink anything after 11 P.M. The next morning, mix the challenge drink according to the instructions provided and drink it before eating or drinking anything else. Carry on with your normal activities for the next six hours, and then collect another urine specimen. Package the specimens according to the kit directions and send them off to the lab. Your health care practitioner will receive the results soon after.

The challenge drink in the intestinal permeability test

contains two different sugars that are water soluble but are not actually metabolized by your body: mannitol and lactulose. Most people readily absorb all or most of the mannitol through the small intestine, but absorb very little of the lactulose. Because mannitol is absorbed but not metabolized, it will later be excreted unchanged in your urine. Because very little lactulose is absorbed through the gut, almost none will be excreted in the urine—it will simply pass through the gut unabsorbed and be excreted in the feces instead. One minor drawback of this test is that some very sensitive patients may have cramping or minor diarrhea from the lactulose.

If you have a leaky gut, however, you will absorb more lactulose than normal through the small intestine, which means that you will excrete more than normal in your urine. If you have an increased lactulose recovery rate—if you have more lactulose than normal in your urine—you may have increased intestinal permeability. If you have an increased mannitol recovery rate—if you excrete it faster than normal in your urine—this too could indicate increased intestinal permeability. If you have a decreased mannitol recovery rate—if you have less mannitol than normal in your urine—it could be because you haven't absorbed as much as normal and the rest was excreted in your feces. This could indicate malabsorption, perhaps because of bacterial overgrowth of the small intestine.

Once you and your health care provider have determined that leaky gut syndrome is the problem, the treatment will depend on the underlying cause of the problem. As we discussed above, one major cause of leaky gut is bacterial overgrowth of the small intestine. Since food allergies and sensitivities are another significant cause of leaky gut syndrome, you might want to investigate these carefully. (See chapter 5 for more information.) Once the bacterial overgrowth is cured or you stop eating the foods that you are sensitive to, your leaky gut problems will start to clear up. Parasites can also sometimes cause leaky gut syndrome (discussed further in chapter 8).

If your leaky gut syndrome is related to prescription medications or over-the-counter nonsteroidal anti-inflammatory drugs (NSAIDs) such as ibuprofen (Advil), aspirin, or naprosyn, discuss alternatives with your doctor. You might be able to reduce the dosage or switch to different drugs.

Traditional Treatments

Diet   Years of eating a poor diet can lead to leaky gut syndrome, especially in older patients. A high-fat, high-sugar diet with too little fiber is often at the root of the problem. Eating a lot of highly processed foods, which often have many additives such as food preservatives and usually have too little fiber, can lead to leaky gut. Patients often improve sharply when they begin to eat a healthier diet. If you have leaky gut syndrome, avoid prepared and processed foods. Eat plenty of fresh vegetables and whole grains; avoid dairy products and fatty foods. Be sure to get plenty of fiber, but avoid too much fruit. Drink at least six to eight glasses of pure water every day. Do not drink alcoholic beverages of any sort.

If you have leaky gut syndrome, it is quite likely that you also have food allergies or intolerances. Your leaky gut syndrome will get better only if you determine which, if any, foods you are sensitive to and avoid those foods. Please refer back to the chapter on food allergies and intolerances for more information.

Alternative Treatments

Other supplements   An underlying cause of leaky gut syndrome is a shortage of the amino acid glutamine. Glutamine is the primary nutrient for the cells that line the small intestine. If you don't get enough glutamine for any of the reasons discussed above, the mucous lining of your small intestine thins out and becomes permeable. Try taking eight grams a day, in capsules or in powder form mixed with water.

As discussed above in the section on dysbiosis, adding friendly bacteria and nutrients to support them is also very helpful for leaky gut syndrome. Rice bran oil, which contains gamma oryzanol, is often helpful for healing leaky gut syndrome. Try taking three 100-milligram capsules daily for four to six weeks. Rice protein concentrate is a good source of healing vitamin E.

Relaxation techniques   Occasional stress often produces mild digestive problems such as heartburn. Prolonged stress, however, can disrupt your digestion so often that you develop leaky gut syndrome. At the least, try to eat nutritious meals in a calm, relaxed, unhurried atmosphere. Chew your food thoroughly. Consider ways to reduce the overall stress level of your life—meditation techniques or yoga, combined with some lifestyle changes and a more relaxed approach to life, may help.

INTESTINAL OBSTRUCTION

If your small intestine is partially or fully blocked for some reason, the chyme will not be able to continue on properly. You'll probably have crampy abdominal pain, nausea, and vomiting; in addition, you may have constipation alternating with bouts of liquid diarrhea. Overall, you will feel very sick—much sicker than if you had intestinal flu or minor food poisoning. Any obstruction of the small intestine is a medical emergency that requires immediate treatment. If you delay getting help, you could develop life-threatening peritonitis (inflammation of the lining of the abdominal wall) or ileus (paralysis of the small intestine).

One common cause of an obstruction in the small intestine is an obstructed or strangulated hernia. In this case, a loop of your intestine has bulged through a gap in your abdominal wall, the flat sheet of muscles that holds your abdominal organs in place. Adhesions, or bands of tissue in the small intestine from previous inflammatory illness or abdominal surgery, can also sometimes cause intestinal obstructions. For unknown reasons, a section of your small intestine can sometimes become twisted, a condition called volvulus. Cancer of the colon can sometimes cause an obstruction of the small intestine. Since cancer of the small intestine is quite rare, it is unlikely to be the cause of an obstruction, but a rare type of growth called a carcinoid can sometimes cause intestinal obstruction. Very rarely, a large, indigestible object such as a swallowed coin will lodge in the small intestine and cause an obstruction.

CHAPTER 7

Gallstones

Your gallbladder is a small, pear-shaped organ, about three to six inches long, that lies beneath your liver in the upper right side of your abdomen. It serves as a reservoir for bile, a greenish-brown digestive fluid made by your liver. When you eat, the gallbladder contracts and releases bile into your small intestine. The bile, which contains cholesterol, bile acids, lecithin, and water, is used to break up and digest fats and to help you absorb vitamins and minerals. Your gallbladder releases about one and half pints of bile every day.

Small tubes called bile ducts connect the gallbladder to the liver and to the small intestine. Sometimes excess cholesterol in your bile forms a tiny crystal that sinks to the bottom of your gallbladder—just as too much sugar in your coffee sinks to the bottom of the cup. Eventually, additional cholesterol adheres to the crystal and forms a gallstone—a small, pebblelike mass. Cholesterol stones account for about 80 percent of all gallstones. Pigment stones, formed from calcium salts, bilirubin, and other natural substances, generally account for the rest. In either case, often more than one stone forms. Gallstones vary considerably in size. Most are well under an inch in diameter, although some are just specks and others can grow to be as large as a small ball. Gallstones grow very slowly—most will remain the same size for years.

Gallstone sludge occurs when many cholesterol crystals accumulate in the gallbladder without ever cohering into a stone. The sludge generally causes no symptoms, but it may occasionally act up.

Gallstones are frequently symptomless and harmless. In fact, about 20 million Americans, or about 10 percent of the population, have gallstones, but most don't even know it. Gallstones and sludge can irritate the gallbladder, however, and sometimes stones are forced into the bile ducts. Symptoms of gallbladder irritation can often mimic those of indigestion or heartburn. In mild cases, an unpleasant sensation of bloating, "fullness," or pressure is the most common symptom; there may also be some slight discomfort or pain in the upper right abdomen. In more serious cases, you will have biliary colic: severe, intermittent pain in the upper right abdomen. The symptoms usually occur a few hours after eating a fatty meal, when the gallbladder contracts to squirt its bile into your small intestine. Often the symptoms go away within an hour or two, as the stone falls back into the gallbladder or is pushed out into the small intestine. Once you start having gallbladder symptoms, however, you are more likely to have them again—and to have them more often.

Sometimes a gallstone is pushed out of the gallbladder during the contraction and gets stuck in the bile duct. The blockage can lead to infection and obstruction of the duct, a condition called acute cholecystitis if the infection is in the gallbladder and cholangitis if the infection is in the bile duct. More rarely, a gallstone will block the bile duct at the entrance to the pancreas and small intestine, causing acute pancreatitis. A blocked bile duct generally causes steady, severe pain in the upper right part of the abdomen, usually along with severe pain in the middle of the abdomen and back (this pain may be mistaken for a heart attack), severe nausea and vomiting, fever and chills, and jaundice (a yellow discoloration of the skin and eyes). A blocked bile duct is a serious and painful problem—get medical attention at once.

If your doctor suspects gallstones, based on your symptoms, he or she may recommend an ultrasound examination to confirm the diagnosis. This is a simple, painless, noninvasive procedure that uses sound waves to create a picture of your gallbladder, bile ducts, and any stones or sludge that may be in them. It is very quick and accurate.

Traditional Treatments

Diet The biggest risk factor for gallstones is being overweight. People who are obese are three to seven times more likely to develop gallstones, even if they have low blood cholesterol levels. On the other hand, crash diets that lead to losing a lot of weight rapidly, or losing weight rapidly and then gaining it back again, can bring on gallstone trouble. If you are overweight and want to avoid gallstones, it's probably best to lose weight sensibly and try to keep it off.

If gallstones contain cholesterol, does that mean a low-cholesterol or low-fat diet can prevent them? The answer is probably not. There's not a lot of evidence to show that a low-fat diet prevents gallstones or that having high blood cholesterol levels causes them. Changing your diet to avoid fatty foods may help prevent or delay a recurrence of gallbladder irritation, but it will not make the gallstones go away once they have formed.

Women, especially as they get older, are more likely to get gallstones than men. There is some evidence to show that women who routinely skip breakfast or just have coffee on an empty stomach are somewhat more likely to get gallstones. So are people who eat a low-fiber, high-sugar diet. Coffee, even decaffeinated, causes gallbladder attacks for some people.

The risk of gallstones increases steadily with age. By the age of sixty, nearly 10 percent of all men and more than 20 percent of all women have them. Other risk factors for gallstones include being pregnant, having a family history of gallstones, using birth control pills or estrogen replacement therapy, and being of Native American ancestry.

If you are at risk for gallstones for any reason, lose weight if you need to. Eating a good breakfast and healthy meals on a regular basis, including foods that are high in fiber—especially fiber from fresh fruits and vegetables, nuts, and beans and legumes—could keep you from developing symptoms. Dietary fiber may help prevent gallstone formation by lowering the acid level of your bile and reducing the amount of deoxycholic acid your body absorbs. Deoxycholic acid is produced by bacteria acting on the bile in your small intestine. It makes cholesterol less soluble in bile, which means the cholesterol is more likely to crystallize in your gallbladder and form stones. A high-fiber diet reduces the amount of deoxycholic acid you produce and also binds the acid and removes it from your body. This could be one reason that vegetarians, who generally eat a lot of fiber, have far fewer gallstones than meat eaters.

Many patients have improved quickly when they changed their diet. One gallbladder patient used to have a sugary pastry and coffee for breakfast, when she ate breakfast at all. When she started having tea, a bowl of oatmeal, and whole wheat toast every morning, she had fewer gallbladder attacks. As a bonus, her improved diet and more regular eating habits helped her lose weight almost effortlessly. A year after losing twenty pounds on her high-fiber diet, she had stopped having gallbladder attacks completely.

Some physicians believe that food allergies are related to gallbladder attacks. Eggs are thought to be a major culprit, but pork, onions, milk, coffee, citrus fruits, corn, beans, and nuts have all been implicated in some cases. If you think your gallbladder attacks are related to a specific food, try an elimination diet as discussed in chapter 5 on food allergies. You may discover that a particular food does relate to your attacks. If it does, you may be able to avoid future attacks by avoiding that food.

Self-help steps   During a mild attack of biliary colic, rest in bed and don't eat (small sips of water are okay). If you have had biliary colic before, your doctor may have prescribed painkillers; take them if you wish. If the pain persists for more than three hours, call your doctor.

Drugs   A drug called ursodiol (Actigall) is usually very helpful for relieving gallbladder symptoms. Ursodiol is a natural bile salt that reduces the amount of cholesterol your liver secretes into the bile; it actually dissolves gallstones and sludge. Most patients need to take the pills for about six months to dissolve the stones completely, although multiple small stones will dissolve more quickly than one large stone. Fortunately, the uncomfortable symptoms of gallstones go away soon after you start taking the medicine.

Surgery Although your gallbladder is an important organ that you should not part with lightly, sometimes removing it is the only way to treat severe gallstones, especially those that block the bile ducts or cause other serious complications. At one time gallbladder surgery meant a large abdominal incision and a long recovery period. Today, gallbladder removal (cholecystectomy) is usually done using advanced laparoscopic surgery techniques that require only a half-inch incision in the abdomen. Requiring a hospital stay of only a day or two, the procedure is safer, less painful, and has a much shorter recovery time than the earlier technique. Laparoscopic surgery is also much easier for older patients—and the older you get, the more likely you are to have gallbladder trouble. Gallbladder surgery is now one of the most common operations in the United States. About 500,000 operations are performed every year; of those, 400,000 are done laparoscopically.

After your gallbladder has been removed, your bile will flow directly from your liver into your small intestine. Generally this has no effect on your digestion and you will have few if any symptoms. Of course, you will no longer have gallbladder discomfort.

An interesting but still experimental approach to large, single gallstones is shock wave lithotripsy. This technique uses sound waves to break up the stone into tiny pieces that can then be dissolved with the drug ursodiol. Gallstones may recur, however. If you are a candidate for lithotripsy, your physician can help you find a medical center that performs it.

Another experimental method for dealing with gallstones is contact dissolution. This procedure involves inserting a needle through the abdomen directly into the gallbladder. An agent that rapidly dissolves the gallstones is instilled over several hours; the needle is then removed. If you are interested in contact dissolution, your physician can help you find a medical center that performs it.

Alternative Treatments

Acupressure/acupuncture   The acupressure/acupuncture points for the gallbladder are on either side of the back of the neck just behind the ears near the base of the skull. Applying pressure here could help relieve gallbladder symptoms.

Reflexology   Working the gallbladder points on your hands and feet may help relieve problems. The hand gallbladder point is on your right hand only, on your palm just below the pad of your ring (fourth) finger. It is a small, round point surrounded by the larger stomach point. Apply fairly strong, steady pressure. The foot gallbladder point is on the sole of your left foot only. It is found toward the outer edge of your foot about halfway between the little toe and your heel. It is a small, round point surrounded by the larger liver point. Apply rotational pressure on the point by pressing the thumb of one hand directly into it and gently rotating the foot in a circular direction with the other hand. Because the gallbladder points are quite small, they may be hard to locate exactly. Applying pressure in the general region will still be helpful, since you will be working not only the gallbladder points but also useful related points.

Herbal therapy   Many traditional herbal remedies are commonly suggested for gallbladder problems. They fall into two broad categories. Cholagogues are herbs that stimulate gallbladder contraction to improve the flow of bile. They may help relieve gallbladder irritation by helping sludge and small stones pass naturally out of the gallbladder. Choleretics are herbs that stimulate the liver to produce bile. They may help prevent gallbladder attacks by improving the solubility of bile, making it less likely that cholesterol will crystallize out.

If you use herbal choleretics, you may have somewhat looser or larger stools than usual due to the increased bile flow. This is normal. If diarrhea develops, however, reduce the dose or stop taking the herb until your bowels are back to normal.

Cholagogues and choleretics should be used *only* as preventive measures for helping to prevent gallbladder irritation. Do not use these herbs to treat an acute gallbladder attack!

Dandelion *(Taraxacum officinale)* is one of the most widely used herbs for the gallbladder. It is known in European, Chinese, and Ayurvedic herbal medicine for its cholagogic and choleretic effects. Different forms of dandelion can be readily found in health food stores. Perhaps the most convenient form is the dried root, ground up and packaged in capsules. The usual recommendation is four grams (eight 500-milligram capsules) three times a day. If you use the liquid extract version, take four to eight milliliters three times a day. For the solid extract version, take 250 to 500 milligrams three times a day. Dandelion has a diuretic effect, so drink plenty of fluids while you take this herb.

Artichoke leaves *(Cynara scolymus)* contain a number of substances, particularly one called cynarin, that have a choleretic effect. Artichoke leaf extract containing about 15 percent cynarin can be purchased at health food stores.

Try taking 500 milligrams three times a day half an hour before meals. Alternatively, you could purchase cynarin tablets. These are more concentrated; take just 500 milligrams a day about half an hour before meals. Artichoke is a mild diuretic; drink extra fluids when taking this herb.

Gentian root *(Gentiana lutea)* is another cholagogue used in traditional European herbal medicine. Gentian is often taken as a tea made by boiling one teaspoon of powdered gentian in half a cup of water for five minutes. Strain before drinking. Try gentian tea half an hour before meals; drink no more than two cups a day.

A South African plant called devil's claw *(Harpago-phytum procumbens)* is sometimes recommended as a cholagogue along the lines of gentian root. Try taking one capsule half an hour before meals. In European herbal medicine, yarrow *(Achillea millefolium)* is also sometimes recommended as a cholagogue. Yarrow is closely related to chamomile and is used for many of the same purposes. Prepare yarrow tea by steeping two tablespoons of the dried herb in one cup of boiling water for ten minutes. Strain before drinking; have half a cup about half an hour before eating. If you are allergic to ragweed, avoid yarrow—it's likely that you are allergic to it as well.

In traditional Ayurvedic medicine, turmeric *(Curcuma longa)* is recommended for its choleretic effect. Turmeric is a bright yellow powder (it is often added to commercial mustards and curry mixes to give them color). To help prevent gallstone symptoms, try taking capsules containing 300 milligrams three times a day. Turmeric may also be helpful for relieving very mild gallstone symptoms, especially the unpleasant bloated or "full" feeling. Do not use it if you are having more severe symptoms—it could actually worsen them.

Milk thistle *(Silybum marianum)*, also called sily-marin, is a very helpful herb for healing and protecting the liver. Because liver function is closely tied to gall-bladder function, silymarin is often helpful for improving the bile flow and making the bile more soluble. Silymarin capsules can be bought at health food stores. Look for a brand that contains 80 percent milk thistle extract. Try swallowing three capsules with a glass of water before every meal to help prevent gallbladder attacks. The dose can be safely raised to as many as six capsules before each meal.

Alfalfa, which is rich in vitamins and minerals, is sometimes recommended by herbalists as a liver cleanser that can also help the gallbladder. If you are having very mild gallbladder symptoms, try taking ten alfalfa tablets with a glass of warm water before meals for two days. Stop taking the tablets and see your doctor if your symptoms get worse during this time or have not improved after two days.

Wild yam tincture is sometimes recommended by herbalists to relieve the symptoms of an acute gallbladder attack. The suggested dose is usually fifteen drops in a glass of warm water, repeated every twenty minutes. While this may give some relief, it is no substitute for immediate medical attention.

Capsules containing peppermint oil are sometimes used by European herbalists to cleanse the gallbladder. There's no evidence that peppermint oil actually does anything, however. Bayberry *(Myrica pensylvanica)* is sometimes recommended as a choleretic by herbalists. The compound myricitrin, found in bayberry, has been shown to stimulate the flow of bile, but other compounds in bayberry have been shown to be carcinogenic. Avoid using bayberry for gallbladder problems. A number of other herbs, including horsetail, catnip, and parsley, are sometimes suggested for gallbladder symptoms. None are likely to be helpful; avoid them.

Vitamin and mineral therapy   Some researchers believe that supplements of vitamin C and vitamin E can help reduce the frequency of gallbladder attacks; vitamin E seems to be the most helpful. Although the connections between vitamins and gallstones is far from proven, you could try taking 1,000 milligrams of vitamin C daily and 300 IU of vitamin E three times a day.

Other supplements   The amino acid taurine is a component of bile acids. Supplemental taurine could help you produce more bile acid, which would help make the cholesterol in your bile more soluble and prevent crystals from forming. It is possible that taking 1,000 milligrams a day of taurine could help prevent the formation of new gallstones. Taurine supplements are available at health food stores.

Lecithin, a fatty substance vital for forming your cell membranes, may also help make cholesterol more soluble. Lecithin is found in egg yolks and some other foods, but the best way to increase your levels is to take supplements of its biologically most active form, phosphatidyl choline. Try capsules up to 500 milligrams daily to help prevent gallstone formation.

Lipotropic supplements are prepared mixtures of herbs and other substances such as phosphatidyl choline that are said to help normalize gallbladder function. Different manufacturers offer varying formulations so if you try different brands, check the instructions on each label.

Some practitioners believe that hypochlorhydria, or a shortage of hydrochloric acid in the stomach, can contribute to the formation of gallstones. Hypochlorhydria can be treated with supplements of hydrochloric acid in the form of glutamic acid hydrochloride (glutamic acid HCL) or betaine hydrochloride with pepsin. Start by taking one capsule with each main meal, then increase the dosage gradually by one capsule to a maximum of three capsules per meal. Cut back if you feel a warm or burning sensation in the stomach, have stomach pain, or feel nauseous. (For more information on hypochlorhydria, see chapter 2.)

Juice therapy   Green juices rich in chlorophyll may help prevent gallbladder attacks. Mix four ounces of pure water with four ounces of alfalfa juice, wheatgrass juice, spinach juice, parsley juice, or other green juice, alone or in combination. Have one or two glasses a day. If you have had a mild gallbladder attack, advocates of juice therapy suggest eating lightly and drinking plenty of pure, organic apple juice, pear juice, and beet juice for several days afterward. This is said to help cleanse the liver and promote the flow of bile. Fennel juice is sometimes suggested to help relieve discomfort from troublesome gallstones. To make fennel juice, remove the feathery leaves and rinse the stems thoroughly. Juice the stems. If you find the anise flavor too strong, add some carrot juice to the mixture. Slowly sip a quarter cup of the fennel juice if gallstone symptoms occur. If the symptoms persist, try another quarter cup.

Hydrotherapy Keeping well hydrated may help prevent gallbladder attacks. If you have gallstones, try drinking six to eight glasses of pure water daily. During a gallbladder attack, drink even more—up to twelve glasses a day.

Homeopathic remedies Very mild gallstone symptoms, especially a "full" feeling or indigestion that occurs several hours after eating, may respond to pulsatilla 6c, taken every ten to fifteen minutes for up to seven doses. Bryonia 6c, taken every ten to fifteen minutes for up to seven doses, may relieve the sensation of food just sitting "like a rock" in your stomach. The tissue salt nat. sulph. 6x, taken every fifteen minutes for up to seven doses, may help relieve discomfort from gallstones.

Liver flush Some health care practitioners suggest a liver flush as a gallstone remedy, although we strongly advise against it. The treatment is said to force troublesome gallstones out of the gallbladder and into the small intestine; the stones are then eliminated. Most formulas for a liver flush involve drinking large amounts of olive oil and lemon juice or grapefruit juice over several days. Some regimens add Epsom salts and other fruit juices to the basic olive oil treatment. People who do liver flushes sometimes find greenish, stonelike masses of varying sizes in their stool, but these are not actually gallstones— they are really conglomerations of the olive oil and lemon juice, along with some other digestive substances that are produced in your intestines. In fact, an olive oil liver flush can be more harmful than helpful. To cope with all the olive oil, your gallbladder will contract to squirt bile into your small intestine. If you have gallstones, however, the contractions may actually force a stone into the bile ducts, where it can lodge and block the duct, with the serious consequences described above.

Combined Treatments

Diet, herbs, vitamins, and lecithin   No dietary or alternative treatment will dissolve existing stones, so the goal of combined treatment is to prevent acute attacks and to slow or stop the formation of additional gallstones. Avoiding fatty foods will help prevent further gallbladder attacks; if coffee triggers an attack for you, avoid it. To help prevent the formation of additional stones, try taking dandelion capsules and lecithin supplements daily. Taking 1,000 milligrams of vitamin C and 300 IU of vitamin E daily may also help prevent stone formation.

If you have an attack of gallbladder pain, get immediate medical attention.

CHAPTER 8

Common Bowel Problems

Your large intestine (also called the bowel) is a muscular tube consisting of two main segments: the colon and the rectum. By far the longest part is the colon. Your colon begins with the cecum, a pouchlike chamber that receives the contents of the small intestine. Your appendix, a small organ filled with lymphatic tissue, is near this juncture, located on the lower right side of your abdomen. After the cecum, the first portion of the colon goes up your right side and is called the ascending colon. The next portion goes across your abdomen under your rib cage and is called the transverse colon. The final portion goes down the left side of your abdomen and is called the descending colon. The contents of the descending colon empty into the rectum and from there are eliminated from the body through the anus. The name large intestine is slightly misleading, since it refers to the wide diameter of the organ, not its length. In all, your colon is about five feet long and about two inches in diameter. Your rectum is about five inches long.

By the time the chyme in your small intestine reaches your colon, most of the nutrients have already been removed and absorbed. What enters your colon consists largely of dietary fiber, indigestible food particles, water, dead bacteria, and lining that has been shed by the small intestine. Within the colon, the chyme will be converted into solid or semisolid feces and then eliminated from the body. In the process, your colon will reabsorb much of the water in the feces into your body.

In this chapter we'll discuss the causes and treatments of three very common colon problems: gas, diarrhea, and constipation. We'll also discuss an often overlooked cause of all three problems: parasites. In the next chapter, we'll discuss bacterial overgrowth of the colon (toxic bowel) and its significant health consequences. We'll also discuss other problems of the large intestine, including Crohn's disease, irritable bowel syndrome, appendicitis, and cancer of the colon. We'll discuss hemorrhoids and other problems of the rectum in chapter 10.

FLATULENCE/GAS

Everyone produces some intestinal gas as a normal byproduct of digestion. In fact, the average person passes gas about fourteen times a day, adding up to a volume of about a quart. Large amounts of gas, however, may be embarrassing or cause uncomfortable bloating and cramping. Generally, flatulence consists mostly of odorless nitrogen, carbon dioxide, and oxygen. Sulfurous foods such as beans add an unpleasant rotten-egg smell. Truly foul-smelling gas is usually caused when bacteria in the colon cause undigested food to ferment, producing small but potent amounts of gases with such evocative names as cadaverine and putrescine. Frequent, foul-smelling gas may be a symptom of constipation, intestinal overgrowth problems, or even parasites (see page 159). As discussed earlier in this book, frequent gas could also be a symptom of lactose intolerance, food allergies or intolerances, pancreatic insufficiency, or dysbiosis.

If your gas pains are unusually severe or prolonged for you, or if they are accompanied by stomach or abdominal pain that continues for more than twenty-four hours, call your doctor.

Traditional Treatments

Diet Some foods do produce more gas when digested than others. Beans are notorious for producing flatulence, chiefly because their skins contain indigestible sugars that pass through the small intestine untouched. When they reach the large intestine, bacteria feast on the sugars and give off large amounts of hydrogen and methane gas as byproducts. That doesn't mean you need to forego beans, which are an excellent, low-calorie, low-fat way to add vegetable protein and nonsoluble fiber to your diet. To cut back on the gas problem, soak dried beans for at least twelve hours in three cups of water for every cup of beans. Drain and rinse well before cooking the beans. If you use convenient, inexpensive canned beans, drain off the liquid and rinse the beans well before eating. Soaking and rinsing removes much of the indigestible sugars in the beans. Don't add baking soda to the beans—it won't help the gas, but it will make the beans hard. If you add beans to your diet gradually, you may notice that the amount of gas will decrease and become less odorous as your intestinal flora adjust. Even so, some gas is inevitable. If you are in a social situation where gas could be embarrassing, it might be best to avoid beans.

Sulfur-containing cruciferous vegetables such as broccoli, Brussels sprouts, cabbage, cauliflower, kale, onions, peas, radishes, and turnips may also give you gas. Cooking these vegetables will help reduce the problem. As with beans, if you gradually start eating these vegetables more often, you will probably have less gas as your intestinal bacteria adjust to the change. Some people find that high-pectin fruits such as apples, apple cider, apricots, blueberries, pears, and bananas give them gas. If this happens to you, try eating fruit before a meal as an appetizer instead of having it as dessert or part of the meal—the pectin will be diluted by the food that follows. If flatulence from fruit persists, cut back on the amounts you eat.

Fermented foods such as yogurt, cheese, sauerkraut, and alcohol give some people gas. If this happens to you, the only real solution is to cut back the amounts you ingest. The artificial sweeteners sorbitol and xylitol may also cause gas in some people. Cut back on your use of these products or stop using them completely if they cause unpleasant gas.

Most people have a few foods that give them gas no matter what. If you know that a particular food creates uncomfortable or embarrassing flatulence for you, it's probably best to avoid it.

Suddenly increasing the amount of fiber in your diet almost always leads to uncomfortable flatulence and bloating. Add fiber to your diet slowly and gradually so that your intestinal flora have time to adjust. If gas occurs, cut back on fiber or add it more slowly.

If you are lactose intolerant and have trouble digesting milk and dairy products, one of the main symptoms will be gas. Food allergies and intolerances also often cause gas. To eliminate the problem, avoid or cut back on foods that you are sensitive to. (See chapter 5, "Food Allergies and Sensitivities," for more information.) Other common causes of intestinal gas are pancreatic insufficiency or dysbiosis. (See chapter 6, "Problems of the Small Intestine," for more information.)

Self-help steps   Stomach gas from drinking carbonated beverages or swallowing air when you eat is usually eliminated by belching, but some of the air passes through the intestines. As with stomach gas, try cutting back on soda pop, seltzer, and beer; give up chewing gum, sucking candies, and smoking. Also try eating more slowly and chewing carefully with your mouth firmly closed.

Drugs   A natural over-the-counter product called Beano can really help prevent gas from beans, broccoli, and other gassy foods. It works by providing the digestive enzyme alpha galactosidase, which digests the sugars in the bean skins. Beano is easy to use—simply sprinkle five or six drops on the first forkful you eat. The liquid has a pleasant taste, slightly like soy sauce. The digestive enzyme is unfortunately destroyed by heat, so don't use Beano in cooking. Beano is readily available in drugstores and health food stores.

Some stomach gas ends up being eliminated through the colon. Discomfort from this and from intestinal gas can be relieved with an over-the-counter drug called simethicone, which helps break up gas bubbles. Simethicone will work best if you chew a couple of tablets after eating. Brand names include Mylicon and Gas-X. Some over-the-counter liquid antacids also contain simethicone. Look for products labeled "antacid/antigas."

Activated charcoal tablets are useful for breaking up and absorbing gas—see the discussion of hydrotherapy below for more information.

Chlorophyll tablets or drops, easily found in pharmacies and health food stores, may help prevent gas. Take the chlorophyll with meals.

Alternative Treatments

Reflexology   Massaging the large intestine points on the soles of your feet and the palms of your hands may help relieve intestinal gas. The large intestine points are located between the arch and the heel, on the inner side of each foot. There are several different points that correspond to the ascending, transverse, descending, and sigmoid colons, but applying steady pressure to the overall area is generally sufficient to provide relief. Two points on your palm correspond to the colon. The first point is about an inch below your fourth finger. The second point, which corresponds more closely with the sigmoid colon, is just above your wrist in line with your third finger. Apply steady pressure by rotating your thumb or a golf ball on the hand points. Repeat as needed.

Chiropractic treatments   Chiropractic adjustment can sometimes relieve persistent gas problems.

Herbal therapy   Herbs that relieve intestinal gas are known as carminatives. Most effective carminatives contain oils that relax the intestinal muscles, which allows the gas to pass through more easily.

The best known and most effective carminative herbs are peppermint, chamomile, anise, caraway, and fennel. If you're having gas, try a cup or two of strong peppermint tea. If you prefer, an alcoholic extract of peppermint (you can get this at a well-stocked pharmacy or health food store) can be used in place of tea; take twenty drops in three ounces of water up to four times a day. Strong chamomile tea is also effective, but be sure you are getting a good product. Purchase whole dried flower heads; avoid powdered or crushed chamomile that may have lost its potency or could be mixed with other, cheaper herbs.

Teas made from caraway, anise, or fennel seeds, which all have a characteristic "licorice" flavor, are safe and effective for relieving gas. Make a tea by crushing a teaspoonful of the seeds and steeping it in one cup of boiling water for fifteen minutes. Strain before drinking.

In traditional Chinese herbal medicine, ginger is recommended for relieving gas. To make ginger tea, steep one teaspoon of freshly grated or finely chopped fresh ginger in one cup of boiling water for ten minutes. Strain before drinking. Tea bags containing dried ginger can be bought at health food stores; these work almost as well as making your own tea from fresh ginger. Capsules containing dried ground ginger are available at health food stores. Try taking one 500-milligram capsule instead of a cup of ginger tea. Additional ginger tea or capsules can be taken as needed.

Ginger is also a gas remedy in traditional Ayurvedic medicine. If you often get gas after eating, try mixing one teaspoon of freshly grated ginger with one teaspoon of freshly squeezed lime juice. To help prevent gas from forming, swallow the mixture as soon as you finish your meal.

Adding garlic, ginger, or nutmeg while cooking foods such as beans or broccoli may help reduce the amount of flatulence they produce. Adding the Asian sea vegetable kombu while the food is cooking is said to help reduce gas.

Juice therapy   Juice made from the fennel stem is as useful for flatulence as tea made from fennel seeds, plus you get some of the abundant dietary fiber found in fennel. To make fennel juice, remove the feathery leaves and rinse the stems thoroughly. Juice the stems. If you find the anise flavor too strong, add some carrot juice to the mixture. To relieve intestinal gas, slowly sip a quarter cup of fresh fennel juice or half a cup of the blend. If the gas persists, try another dose. This remedy helps the gas pass more quickly, but does not reduce the quantity of it.

Green juices rich in chlorophyll may also help relieve flatulence. Mix four ounces of pure water with four ounces of alfalfa juice, wheatgrass juice, spinach juice, parsley juice, or other green juice, alone or in combination. Have no more than two glasses a day.

Hydrotherapy   Activated charcoal, easily available at health food stores and well-stocked pharmacies, is often very helpful for relieving flatulence. Mix two to three tablespoons of activated charcoal with one ounce of cool water in a twelve-ounce glass. When the mixture is well blended, slowly stir in enough water to fill the glass. Sip the mixture through a straw. Alternatively, swallow two activated charcoal tablets with a glass of water. Activated charcoal absorbs the gas and is useful for reducing odor problems. Use activated charcoal only occasionally—frequent use can lead to impaired digestion and could interfere with any other medications you take.

Homeopathic remedies   Which homeopathic remedy you choose for flatulence will depend on your symptoms. If your stomach feels bloated and full of gas, try argentum nit. 6c every half hour; repeat up to four doses. If the gas feels "stuck" in your intestines or you have a lot of rumbling, try lycopodium 6c every half hour; repeat up to ten doses. For gas and indigestion from a food that disagrees with you, try carbo vegetabilis 6c every fifteen minutes for up to seven doses. For a sudden attack of gas, try carbo vegetabilis 6c; repeat every thirty minutes as needed up to ten doses. Gas accompanied by mild nausea might be relieved by sepia 6c taken every thirty minutes up to seven doses.

Relaxation techniques   You will have less gas if you swallow less air when you eat. Gulping your food is a common cause of stomach gas, some of which will be passed through the colon. Try to have your meals in a pleasant, relaxed environment. Eat slowly and chew each mouthful thoroughly. Yoga exercises that help tone the digestive system and abdominal area may help. The knee-squeeze and shoulder-stand exercises are particularly helpful. Directions for these exercises can be found in any good book on yoga techniques.

Combined Treatments

Diet and hydrotherapy   By gradually building up your tolerance for some gas-producing foods and avoiding others, you can reduce the amount of gas you pass. If uncomfortable gas does occur, activated charcoal, especially in the convenient tablet form, is quite effective for relieving the discomfort and reducing the odor.

Diet and herbs or juice   By gradually building up your tolerance for some gas-producing foods and avoiding others, you can reduce the amount of gas you pass. If uncomfortable gas does occur, herbal remedies such as strong fennel or ginger tea often help relieve the discomfort by helping the gas pass more quickly. Fennel juice also helps the gas pass quickly.

DIARRHEA

Occasional diarrhea—the frequent, urgent passing of loose, watery stools—is a very common digestive problem. In most cases, it's simply your body's efficient, if unpleasant, way of getting rid of germs, toxins, or food that disagrees with you.

Often diarrhea is caused by a bacterial infection (gastroenteritis and traveler's diarrhea are in this category) or by a virus. Diarrhea from these causes is sometimes referred to as intestinal flu, twenty-four-hour flu, or stomach bug; traveler's diarrhea, especially if it results from travel outside the country, is sometimes called turista or Montezuma's revenge. No matter what it's called, you have secretory diarrhea, because toxins from the microbes cause the cells lining your colon to secrete more fluid than they absorb—the opposite of what they are supposed to do. Generally these ailments are minor and self-limiting. You feel lousy for a day or two, and then recover completely. In such cases, the simple treatments discussed below will usually help relieve the discomfort and may help you get back to normal more quickly.

Diarrhea can also be caused by what you eat or by overeating. In this case, the cells lining your colon can't absorb all the fluid in your stool and you have osmotic diarrhea, so called because the fluid balance through the membrane is disrupted. Overeating, especially of foods that are very spicy, high in fiber, very fatty, or high in sugar, is the most common cause of osmotic diarrhea. Generally no treatment is necessary—you'll feel a lot better as soon as the offending food has left your system. Food allergies, lactose intolerance, and overuse of magnesium-containing antacids can also cause osmotic diarrhea.

If you have frequent bouts of diarrhea, you may have a more serious problem that should be investigated thoroughly with your health care provider. Frequent diarrhea can cause nutritional deficiencies and leave you open to problems such as intestinal overgrowth. Possible causes of frequent diarrhea include parasites, bacterial overgrowth, irritable bowel syndrome, and Crohn's disease (see chapter 9), food allergies and intolerances (see chapter 5), and dysbiosis in the small intestine (see chapter 6).

The loss of fluids from diarrhea can be very serious for infants, children, chronically ill people or people with impaired immune systems, and the elderly. Be alert for the symptoms of dangerous dehydration: weakness, dry mouth, restlessness, extreme thirst, little or no urination. Dehydration from diarrhea needs immediate medical attention.

For healthy adults, diarrhea that doesn't go away in a few days, is accompanied by a high fever or abdominal tenderness, contains blood, or recurs often can be a sign of a more serious problem. Call your doctor. If your diarrhea is so severe or continues for so long that you lose more than 4 percent of your total body weight within a week or less (for example, more than six pounds if you weigh 150 pounds), call your doctor.

Traditional Treatments

Diet Since diarrhea is your body's way of getting rid of something undesirable, we suggest you go with the flow, as it were, unless there is reason for concern. Instead of trying to stop the diarrhea, try to replace the fluids your body loses. You need to drink a lot of liquid—at least eight and preferably twelve eight-ounce glasses a day while your diarrhea lasts. Clear liquids and diluted, unsweetened fruit juices are good; so is flavored gelatin. Plain water is always good, as is weak, unsweetened tea or strained vegetable juices. Some people find that clear broths or sports drinks are helpful. Avoid alcohol, sweetened drinks, and anything containing milk (milk shakes or ice cream, for example).

Diarrhea makes you lose electrolytes (chemicals such as potassium that your body needs in order to maintain proper functioning) along with fluid. To replace the electrolytes, in a large glass combine eight ounces of apple, orange, or other fruit juice with half a teaspoon of honey and a pinch of ordinary table salt. In another large glass, combine eight ounces of plain water and a quarter teaspoon of baking soda (sodium bicarbonate). Sip from each glass alternately. The fruit juice contains the potassium you need, while the salt and baking soda provide the necessary sodium. The sugar from the fruit juice and honey helps you absorb the electrolytes better.

You probably won't feel much like eating anyway, but it's usually best to avoid food until the worst of the diarrhea is over. Once you've gone several hours without a bout, or if your stool seems to be getting back to normal, you'll probably also be feeling better and will want to think about food again.

While you're recovering from an attack of diarrhea, we suggest you eat several small meals spread throughout the day rather than one or two big meals. Try having something that is thick, starchy, and not too sweet. Blenderized chicken soup with rice, cream of wheat, oatmeal, plain baked potatoes (no butter), bananas, tapioca pudding, and the like are all easily digested and won't irritate your bowel further. We usually suggest going on the

BRAT diet—bananas, rice, applesauce, and toast—for a day or two. The pectin in the apples and bananas helps relieve your symptoms and normalize your stool.

Until your digestion is fully back to normal, avoid fatty or fried foods, sugary foods, carbonated beverages, gas-producing foods such as cabbage and beans, and dairy products such as milk, cottage cheese, and ice cream. All these foods are hard to digest and will only irritate your system.

Sometimes diarrhea is caused by artificial sweeteners such as sorbitol, mannitol, or xylitol, which are often used in dietetic baked goods, candies, and chewing gum. Sorbitol is found naturally in high-pectin fruits such as apples, bananas, pears, and grapes and in juices made from these fruits. If natural sorbitol or artificial sweeteners give you diarrhea, avoid foods containing them.

Diarrhea is often caused by overeating or eating foods that upset your digestion. If you overeat, especially if you eat too many sweets, diarrhea may be the price you pay. Once the offending foods have passed through your system, you should quickly feel better. If you are lactose intolerant, dairy products could be causing your diarrhea—avoid these foods in the future. Your diarrhea may be caused by a food intolerance or food allergy. To avoid future problems, you need to identify and avoid the food(s). (For more information, see chapter 5, "Food Allergies and Sensitivities.")

Self-help steps   Frequent doses of nonprescription liquid antacids containing magnesium hydroxide can cause diarrhea. If your antacid is giving you diarrhea, consider switching to a nonprescription H_2 blocker instead such as Zantac. (See chapter 2, "Heartburn and Indigestion," for more information.) High doses of vitamin C (more than

2,000 milligrams a day) can also cause diarrhea. If you take supplemental vitamin C, try cutting back. Antibiotic drugs such as penicillin or tetracycline can cause diarrhea, because they also kill the useful bacteria in your digestive tract. If you think a course of antibiotics has caused your diarrhea, try eating some live-culture yogurt or taking acidophilus tablets (see the section on bacterial overgrowth in chapter 9 for more information). If the diarrhea persists or if you need to take antibiotics frequently, discuss a change of medication with your doctor.

If your diarrhea is from an illness (intestinal flu or the like), you may be able to avoid infecting the people around you by frequently washing your hands (especially after a bowel movement), not sharing any glasses or eating utensils, and disinfecting the toilet after every use.

To help prevent traveler's diarrhea, be very careful about what you eat and drink when visiting a foreign country, especially in underdeveloped regions of the world. Eat only cooked foods; peel all fruits and eat only cooked vegetables (no salads or fruit cups). Especially in tropical climates, try to avoid meat, raw fish, and dairy products. Only drink water or other beverages that are bottled or boiled. Do not add ice to drinks. Avoid eating food from street vendors. Sometimes traveler's diarrhea is not from unfamiliar germs in food or water but simply from the stress and changes of travel; altitude changes and jet lag are often to blame. In such cases, your digestion will return to normal as soon as your body adjusts. Sometimes certain drugs you take as part of your travel—antimalarial medications, sleeping pills, antacids—cause the problem. Once your body has a chance to adjust, you probably won't need sleep aids and the like, and your diarrhea will go away. If you must take disease-preventive drugs, discuss possible side effects and how to treat them with your doctor when the drugs are prescribed.

Drugs Numerous over-the-counter medicines for relieving diarrhea symptoms are found in pharmacies. Diarrhea is your body's way of getting rid of toxins, however, so taking these medicines may actually keep you from getting better. In addition, many of the most popular antidiarrheal drugs have not been shown to be particularly effective, although for most people they are safe to take.

There are times, however, when diarrhea is extremely inconvenient and you may temporarily need one of these medicines. We generally recommend a formulation that contains loperamide (Imodium or its generic equivalent). This drug slows the action of the intestines and is usually effective within one to two hours. Take loperamide only if your diarrhea is from an illness. Don't take it if you have inflammatory bowel disease or irritable bowel syndrome or if your diarrhea has been caused by antibiotic treatment or overindulgence.

Another effective nonprescription treatment for diarrhea is polycarbophil (Equalactin, FiberCon, Mitrolan, or the generic equivalent). Chewable polycarbophil tablets help to absorb water and solidify the bowel movement.

Many nonprescription diarrhea medications contain adsorbents such as activated attapulgite. Although medications such as Donnagel, Kaopectate, and Rheaban or their generic equivalents are safe, they are not particularly effective. The one adsorbent formulation that is often helpful is pink bismuth (Pepto-Bismol or the generic equivalent). Pink bismuth does help relieve the symptoms of mild diarrhea. More usefully, it helps prevent and treat traveler's diarrhea. If you will be traveling to a place where hygiene is a concern, begin taking a tablespoonful or tablet of pink bismuth with meals one full day before you leave. Continue to take the pink bismuth during your trip and for two days after your return—but to avoid possible problems don't take it continuously for more than three weeks. Pink bismuth causes a harmless, temporary blackening of the stool. Constipation is a possible side effect. The salicylate in pink bismuth may cause a ringing in your ears. If this happens, cut back on your dose until the ringing goes away.

Many over-the-counter antidiarrheal drugs claim to relieve the uncomfortable cramps that usually accompany diarrhea. Although these formulas do contain drugs that are capable of relieving cramping, they do not contain them in amounts large enough to be helpful.

In more serious cases of diarrhea, prescription medications may be needed. Drugs combining diphenoxylate and atropine (Lomotil, Diphenatol, Lomanate, or the generic equivalent) are quite effective. If you are planning a trip to a place where traveler's diarrhea is a possibility, ask your doctor to prescribe some such medication for you in advance. However, you should be aware that diphenoxylate with atropine has side effects that can make some chronic conditions worse. Your doctor will probably not prescribe it if you have inflammatory bowel disease or irritable bowel syndrome; emphysema, asthma, or any other chronic lung disease; an enlarged prostate; or gallstones. It is very dangerous to take diphenoxylate and atropine along with monoamine oxidase (MAO) inhibitors such as Nardil, Marplan, Furuxone, Parnate, and related drugs. Severe side effects can occur, even if you have not taken the MAO inhibitor for several days. Diphenoxylate and atropine should not be taken along with some other prescription medications, including antibiotics, central nervous system (CNS) depressants, and tricyclic antidepressants (Elavil, Anafranil, and similar drugs).

If you will be traveling, you could also ask your doctor about taking preventive doses of the antibiotic doxycycline (Doxy-Caps, Vibramycin, or the equivalent generic). This long-acting type of tetracycline may help keep you healthy, but it will also make your skin much more sensitive to sunlight. Take doxycycline with food or milk to avoid upsetting your stomach. While you are taking this drug, do not take antacids, calcium supplements, iron supplements, and vitamins containing iron within two to three hours of your dose.

An alternative to doxycycline is trimethoprim with sulfamethoxazole (Bactrim, Sulfaprim, Triazole or the generic equivalent), which works well and causes a little less sensitivity to sun. On the other hand, this is a more potent drug that can cause blood problems. This drug should be taken with a full glass of water; it is important not to miss any doses.

Prescription drugs that contain opium or paregoric are very effective for stopping diarrhea. They work by slowing the action of the intestines, which reduces cramping and allows excess water to be reabsorbed rather than excreted. Opiates are usually effective within two to six hours. The amount of opium in these medications is quite small and does not have a narcotic effect, but it may make you groggy.

Alternative Treatments

Acupressure/acupuncture The traditional acupressure points for diarrhea are conception vessel 6, which is located on your abdomen just below your navel; stomach meridians 13, which are located on both sides of your abdomen just above the hips; and stomach meridians 36, which are located on each leg on the front just below the knee. Applying gentle pressure on these points may help relieve diarrhea symptoms, especially cramping.

Reflexology Massaging the large intestine points on the soles of your feet and the palms of your hands may help relieve diarrhea symptoms, especially cramping. The large intestine points are located between the arch and the heel, on the inner side of each foot. There are several different points that correspond to the ascending, transverse, descending, and sigmoid colons, but applying steady pressure to the overall area is generally sufficient to provide relief. Two points on your palm correspond to the colon. The first point is about an inch below your fourth finger. The second point, which corresponds more closely with the sigmoid colon, is just above your wrist in line with your third finger. Apply steady pressure by rotating your thumb or a golf ball on the hand points. Repeat as needed.

Herbal therapy Dried (not fresh) blueberries are a traditional European remedy for diarrhea; they can help relieve symptoms. Soak a teaspoonful or so of the berries (available in health food stores and well-stocked grocery stores) in one cup of boiling water until the berries are softened, about five minutes. Drink the liquid and then eat the berries. Repeat three to seven times daily. The tannins and pectin in the blueberries are what make this remedy effective. Tannins help reduce intestinal inflammation, while pectin helps absorb water and slow the transit time for the stool.

Teas made from blackberry, raspberry, or blueberry leaves, from blackberry root, and from wood betony or lady's-mantle are helpful because they too are high in tannin—and they also help replace the fluid that you're losing. Use one to two teaspoons of leaves to one cup of boiling water. Let steep for ten to fifteen minutes before drinking. If you use blackberry root, let it steep for twenty minutes. Drink no more than six cups a day. If you want to try raspberry leaf tea, be sure to purchase exactly that at the health food store—don't purchase raspberry-flavored black tea or herbal mixes that contain only a small amount of raspberry leaves or raspberry flavoring.

Goldenseal is often recommended by herbalists as a remedy for diarrhea. Goldenseal contains an alkaloid called berberine, which has been shown to inhibit the function of diarrhea-causing microbes and parasites. To make an infusion of goldenseal, steep two teaspoons of dried goldenseal root in one cup of boiling water for fifteen minutes. Strain and drink. Take no more than three cups a day. If you prefer capsules, try 500 to 1,000 milligrams of the freeze-dried root three times a day. In liquid form, use one to two teaspoons of the tincture or half a teaspoon of the fluid extract three times a day. Many people mix the fluid with water or fruit juice.

Tea made from barberry (also called Oregon grape) is a Native American remedy for diarrhea. Avoid using bayberry bark (which is not related to barberry)—it has so much tannin that it is potentially dangerous.

Weak teas made from peppermint, chamomile, and

other mild herbs are a good way to get the fluids you need while you have diarrhea.

Other supplements Some practitioners believe that eating live-culture yogurt or taking supplements of friendly bacteria such as *Lactobacillus acidophilus* or *Lactobacillus bulgaricus* can help relieve diarrhea. Although this may help in cases of diarrhea from antibiotics, it generally doesn't do much for diarrhea from illness. In fact, the yogurt may be hard to digest and could make your symptoms worse. Once your diarrhea subsides, however, live-culture yogurt or lactobacilli supplements can help your digestion return to normal more quickly by helping to restore a good balance of bacteria in your intestines. (See the discussion of intestinal overgrowth in chapter 9 for more information.)

Juice therapy In traditional Ayurvedic medicine, pomegranate juice is used to treat diarrhea. It's much easier to buy bottled pomegranate juice at your health food store than it is to try to make your own. If you can't find the unsweetened kind, cut the juice with equal amounts of water. Otherwise, the added sugar could make your diarrhea worse.

Hydrotherapy Activated charcoal, easily available at health food stores and well-stocked pharmacies, may help relieve diarrhea, particularly traveler's diarrhea. Mix two to three tablespoons of activated charcoal with one ounce of cool water in a twelve-ounce glass. When the mixture is well blended, slowly stir in enough water to fill the glass. Sip the mixture through a straw. Alternatively, swallow two activated charcoal tablets with a glass of water.

Homeopathy Which homeopathic remedy you should try depends on your symptoms. For diarrhea with nausea and vomiting, with chills, or for traveler's diarrhea, try arsen. alb. 6c once every hour for up to ten doses. Diarrhea with lots of rumbling and cramps may be helped by pulsatilla 6c once every hour for up to ten doses. For diarrhea from overeating or eating foods that disagree with you, try aloe 6c once every hour for up to ten doses.

Combined Treatments

Diet and herbal teas The best treatment for diarrhea is to drink plenty of clear liquids. Astringent herbal teas made from raspberry leaves or other herbs are a good source of liquids and may also help relieve intestinal discomfort.

CONSTIPATION

Despite the common belief that a daily bowel movement is essential to good health, the normal frequency of bowel movements varies widely from person to person. Some have several movements a day, while others may defecate as infrequently as three times a week. Medically speaking, you are constipated or "irregular" only if you have fewer movements than you normally do, or if your stool is hard, dry, and difficult to pass. If you are constipated, you will probably feel bloated, uncomfortable, and sluggish; you may also have a dull headache and intestinal cramps.

Along with many other health care providers today, we feel that bowel transit time—the length of time it takes for food to move through your digestive system, from your mouth to elimination in the stool—is a far better measure of good bowel function than simply counting the number of movements. Slow bowel transit time allows your colon to reabsorb too much water, which makes the stool dry and hard to pass. Slow bowel transit time also allows your colon to reabsorb wastes and toxins that should be quickly eliminated instead. As we'll discuss more completely in the section on bowel toxicity in the next chapter, the longer your stool remains in your bowel, the more likely it is that the bacteria there will give off toxins that could cause bowel diseases such as colon cancer.

To measure your own bowel transit time, start by eating a marker food and noting the exact time. The food should be something that will be easily visible in your stool later on. Corn kernels are a popular choice; beets will turn your stool a deep magenta color. If you prefer, swallow five or six activated charcoal tablets—these will turn your stool black. Note the exact time when the marker food first appears in your stool and when it last appears.

If you are eating a good, nutritious diet, your transit time will probably be between eighteen and twenty-four hours. If your transit time is longer than that, you almost certainly need more fiber, more water, and more exercise. We urge you to make the dietary and self-help steps below part of your daily life.

Constipation is almost always caused by too little fiber, too little water, and too little exercise—singly or in combination. Sometimes, however, a medication can cause constipation. Iron or calcium supplements, aluminum-based antacids, some antidepressants, some painkillers (particularly codeine), and some high blood pressure drugs are common culprits. If you think a drug is causing your constipation, and increasing the amount of fiber and liquid you consume doesn't help, discuss the problem with your doctor. You may be able to switch to a different drug or a lower dose. Prolonged bed rest or inactivity can also cause constipation. Premenstrual or pregnant women often become constipated as their hormone levels change; constipation is a common symptom of premenstrual stress (PMS). Constipation is also a problem for people with degenerative nerve diseases such as multiple sclerosis or Parkinson's disease.

Occasional constipation is normal and happens to almost everyone. If you also notice blood in your stool or if you also have severe abdominal pain or a high fever, call your doctor. A change in your usual bowel habits could indicate a medical problem. If you start having frequent constipation on your normal diet, or if your stool is narrower than usual, call your doctor, especially if you are over the age of forty.

Traditional Treatments

Diet   Too little fiber in the diet is almost always the root cause of constipation, and adding fiber is almost always the best treatment. (For more on the importance of fiber, see the next chapter.) A fiber-rich diet, combined with plenty of liquids, will relieve constipation and help keep it from recurring. If you are often constipated, look carefully at your diet. You probably eat a lot of processed or prepared foods, dairy products, and sugar. You probably don't eat many fruits or vegetables or whole grains. If you're like an average American, you eat only fifteen to twenty grams of fiber every day and have a bowel transit time of forty-eight hours or longer. To prevent constipation (and to get many other health benefits as well), increase your fiber intake to at least thirty or thirty-five grams every day. You can do this easily by eating two to four servings of fruit, and three to five servings of vegetables, every day. Add one or two servings of whole grains such as whole wheat bread, oatmeal, or bran cereal, and you'll be up to thirty grams a day easily. A single serving of oatmeal at breakfast, for example, gives you nearly three grams of fiber, has only about a hundred calories, and gets your day off to a good, nutritious start. A slice of pumpernickel bread has about four grams of fiber, while a slice of white bread has less than one. Add fiber to your diet gradually—suddenly adding a lot can lead to bloating, gassiness, diarrhea, and other problems.

Drinking plenty of liquids is another easy step toward eliminating constipation. Six to eight glasses a day will do a lot to relieve it. Plain water—free, noncaloric, having no side effects—is ideal. Avoid more than a glass or two of milk each day. Limit fruit juices to just one or two glasses a day—they are high in calories and the sorbitol in apple juice, grape juice, and pear juice could cause diarrhea.

Sometimes patients are very reluctant to make the dietary changes needed to add substantial amounts of fiber to their diet. In such cases, we recommend adding a single unpeeled apple a day to the diet. Most patients find that even this small amount of additional fiber helps their constipation problem. An average apple contains about eighty calories and about two grams of fiber. Most of the fiber is water-soluble pectin, which helps keep stools soft and easily passed.

The traditional dietary remedy for constipation is prunes or prune juice. Dried apricots or figs are also popular. Dried fruits do contain goodly amounts of helpful fiber. The fruits and prune juice also contain isatin, a natural laxative, which is what really makes them effective for regularity. You should get results within twenty-four hours.

Sometimes a cup of coffee, which is a mild natural laxative, is all you need.

Self-help steps   Resisting the urge to defecate is a very common cause of constipation. If you feel the urge, respond to it. Take the time to have a full evacuation. Try to have a bowel movement at about the same time every day, preferably in the morning after breakfast. If your family schedule in the morning is just too hectic for a few minutes of privacy in the bathroom, find another time, again preferably after a meal. Food entering your stomach stimulates the colon to contract. You want to take advantage of this natural action to "train" your bowel. At first you may need some extra time to produce a movement, but within a couple of weeks on a regular schedule you should be able to defecate quickly and fully. Until then, take your time. Some patients find that having something hot to drink (a cup of coffee is good, since coffee is also a mild laxative) followed immediately by something cold (your morning orange juice would be good) helps to stimulate a bowel movement.

Getting more exercise often helps frequent constipation. Simply going for a twenty-minute walk every day tones the abdominal muscles and stimulates the intestines. If you can't get out for a walk, doing any sort of mild exercise that moves the abdominal muscles—toe touches, for example—will help.

Drugs   Every year Americans spend over $700 million on laxatives. A wide variety of nonprescription laxatives can be found in any drugstore, but doctors generally suggest these only for occasional constipation that has not been helped by more dietary fiber and liquids in the diet. Once regularity returns, stop using the laxative—frequent use of laxatives can cause your intestines to become "lazy," so that you become dependent on the drug to move your bowels. Laxatives can also interfere with any medications you may be taking. In general, it's advisable to avoid taking a laxative within two hours of taking another medication.

Some laxatives can cause foods to move through your intestines so rapidly that the nutrients can't be absorbed by your body. Because of this, laxatives can sometimes be abused as a form of weight control and as part of the pattern of purging behavior known as bulimia. The serious consequences of laxative abuse include diarrhea, colon disease, and liver disease.

Laxatives come in many forms: liquid, capsule, emulsion, tablet, suppository, granules, syrup, powder, wafers, chewable tablets, and even chewing gum. They fall into several basic categories: bulk forming; emollient; lubricant; stimulant; stimulant/emollient combinations; and saline.

Of all the possible laxatives, health care providers much prefer that you use the bulk-forming kind, because these laxatives cause responses that most naturally resemble the way your body works. Bulk-forming laxatives contain natural or synthetic fiber in the form of polysaccharides and cellulose derivatives such as calcium polycarbophil (Equalactin, Fiberall, FiberCon or the generic equivalent), methylcellulose (Citrucel or the generic equivalent), or psyllium (Fiberall, Konsyl, Metamucil or the generic equivalent). Also sometimes called "vegetable" or "natural" laxatives, bulk-forming laxatives absorb water and form a soft gel in your colon, which helps your stool pass easily. Always take bulk-forming laxatives with a full eight-ounce glass of water, fruit juice, or other fluid. To avoid gas, bloating, and diarrhea from suddenly adding a lot of fiber to your system, start with small amounts (about a teaspoon) and gradually increase the dose over several days. If you use the powdered form, be sure to stir the mixture well and drink it all immediately. Results usually occur in twelve to twenty-four hours, but may take longer for some people. Bulk-forming laxatives can be used safely over long periods of time, but it is certainly more interesting and convenient to simply eat more fiber as part of your daily diet.

Almost all emollient laxatives contain docusate, which helps to soften the fecal mass and make it easier to pass. Among the many brands available are Colace, Dialose, Diocto, Disonate, Regutol, and Therac Plus; the generic equivalent will work just as well. Emollients are often helpful if you have been constipated for several days. Your doctor may recommend using an emollient if you should avoid straining for a bowel movement, particularly following surgery or a heart attack or when elimination is painful due to hemorrhoids or other physical problems. Although most of our patients prefer taking capsules, emollients are also available as liquids and syrups. Results usually occur in twelve to seventy-two hours. Use emollient laxatives only for short-term treatment; don't take them for longer than a week.

Lubricant laxatives contain mineral oil, which coats and softens the fecal mass and allows it to pass easily. However, mineral oil can cause serious side effects such as malabsorption and bowel incontinence. Use mineral oil only if your doctor recommends it. Castor oil should never be used to treat constipation.

Stimulant laxatives are effective in the treatment of constipation, especially if you have not moved your bowels for several days, but they often cause cramping, griping, and the passing of excessive amounts of fluid. Even worse, they don't help your bowel return to normal function. Take a stimulant laxative only if your health care provider recommends it.

Most stimulant laxatives contain bisacodyl (Carter's Little Pills, Dulcolax), cascara sagrada, phenolphthalein (Ex-Lax, Modane, Unilax), or senna. Although cascara sagrada and senna are plant-based laxatives that have been recommended by herbalists for centuries, they are no more "natural" than any other stimulant laxative and are no more pleasant to use. (We'll discuss these two laxatives further in the herbal therapy section below.)

Results from stimulant laxatives usually occur in six to twelve hours; the effects of one dose can last for up to three days. Use stimulant laxatives with caution and only if bulk-forming laxatives have given you no relief. Women who are pregnant or nursing should avoid stimulant laxatives; use bulk-forming laxatives instead. Do not use stimulant laxatives for more than one week. Laxatives containing phenolphthalein harmlessly discolor your urine and feces in colors ranging from pink to red. Do not use laxatives containing senna or phenolphthalein if you also take a diuretic or high blood pressure medication. Do not take antacids with a laxative containing phenolphthalein.

In an effort to make the effects of stimulant laxatives less uncomfortable, many manufacturers make combined stimulant/emollient formulations such as Correctol and

Feen-A-Mint. As with stimulants, use these mixtures with caution.

Saline laxatives (sometimes called purgatives) are those that use some form of chemical salt, such as magnesium citrate (also known as citrate of magnesia), magnesium hydroxide (also known as milk of magnesia), magnesium sulfate (also known as Epsom salts), or sodium biphosphate (the active ingredient in some prepared enemas) to stimulate a rapid and complete bowel movement. These laxatives are not meant for the treatment of simple constipation. Rather, they are used to evacuate the bowel, particularly in preparation for certain diagnostic procedures such as a colonoscopy. Follow the instructions of your physician regarding any dietary restrictions and how much and when to take the laxative. Saline laxatives are usually taken in liquid form, although tablets and enemas are sometimes recommended. Results usually occur in thirty minutes to three hours.

Sometimes a simple glycerin suppository can stimulate a bowel movement; do not, however, use suppositories that contain anything else. In severe cases, you may need to relieve your constipation with a simple enema. You can purchase inexpensive prepared enema solutions in any drugstore (Fleet is a popular brand); follow the instructions on the package. If you prefer to prepare your own enema, use only plain lukewarm water; do not add soapsuds, herbs, Epsom salts, or anything else. Use no more than two cups of water. High colonics, colonic irrigation, and other "colon cleansing" enemas should be avoided. These enemas can cause serious depletion of the friendly bacteria in your colon and can also deplete electrolytes.

Alternative Treatments

Acupressure/acupuncture   An acupressure technique that often helps relieve mild constipation is to apply pressure to a point on your abdomen halfway between your navel and pubic bone. Lie flat on your back on a firm surface and place the fingertips of one hand on the point. Press down firmly and hold for thirty seconds. Repeat five more times.

A trained acupuncturist will release energy along the conception vessel meridian on your abdomen between your navel and pubic bone, an area also known as the Sea of Energy.

Reflexology   Massaging the large intestine points on the soles of your feet and the palms of your hands may help relieve mild constipation. The large intestine points are located between the arch and the heel, on the inner side of each foot. There are several different points that correspond to the ascending, transverse, descending, and sigmoid colons, but applying steady pressure to the overall area is generally sufficient to provide relief. Two points on your palm correspond to the colon. The first point is about an inch below your fourth finger. The second point, which corresponds more closely with the sigmoid colon, is just above your wrist in line with your third finger. Apply steady pressure by rotating your thumb or a golf ball on the hand points. Repeat as needed.

Massaging the liver point on the tops of your feet may also help constipation, especially if you feel bloated or "clogged." This point is found between the big and second toes just below the bottom joint.

Chiropractic treatments   Chiropratic adjustment can sometimes relieve persistent constipation.

Herbal therapy Herbal remedies that add natural fiber are a good way to help constipation. Unsweetened breakfast cereals that contain large amounts of bran—the fibrous outer coating of grains such as wheat, oats, corn, or rice—are a good approach. These cereals are readily available in health food stores and grocery stores. If you prefer, purchase pure bran and sprinkle a few teaspoons on your regular breakfast cereal. As a bonus, bran, especially rice bran and oat bran, may help reduce your blood cholesterol levels.

Psyllium, the ingredient found in many bulk-forming laxatives such as Metamucil, is made from the husks of the tiny seeds of the plantago plant (also called plantain). Psyllium seeds, sometimes called fleaseeds, are sold in well-stocked health food stores, sometimes under the slightly misleading name of natural vegetable powder. To use psyllium, stir a small amount (about a teaspoon) into an eight-ounce glass of water or juice; drink all the mixture immediately. Results usually occur in twelve to twenty-four hours.

Flaxseeds are very useful remedies for constipation. These seeds contain large amounts of the water-soluble fiber mucilage, which helps make the stool soft, bulky, and easy to pass. Stir a tablespoon of the seeds into an eight-ounce glass of water and let the mixture stand for several hours or overnight before drinking. Have no more than three glasses a day. You should get results within twenty-four hours. If you prefer, you can make a tasty blenderized drink by mixing the soaked flaxseeds with fruit juice, yogurt, bananas, and the like. Powdered flaxseed, can be mixed with water or juice and drunk immediately or it can be added to blender drinks or sprinkle it on yogurt or breakfast cereal; it is available at health food stores. Since flaxseed is high in oil, select a defatted variety that won't go rancid.

Slippery elm bark is a useful herbal remedy that acts as a bowel lubricant. Try stirring two teaspoons of powdered bark into a glass of water or juice.

If bulk-forming laxatives don't help your constipation, an herbalist may suggest using a stimulant herb such as cascara sagrada bark, buckthorn bark, or senna. These herbs contain anthraquinones, which cause your lower intestine to absorb less water from the stool. Cascara sagrada is made from the dried bark of a small tree found in the Pacific Northwest; buckthorn is botanically very similar to cascara and is also made from the bark of the plant. Over-the-counter preparations of cascara bark (Nature's Remedy is a popular brand) are usually in the form of a liquid extract with some flavoring added to disguise the extremely bitter taste. The usual dosage is very small—just half a teaspoon of the extract is effective. Even this amount can cause intestinal griping and diarrhea. Capsules and pills containing the powdered bark are also available. Herbalists who prepare their own mixtures usually age the bark for at least a year to reduce its potency.

Senna, also known as cassia, is the active ingredient in some nonprescription constipation remedies such as Senokot. Senna should be used cautiously in small doses, since it is a fairly potent laxative that can cause painful griping and nausea; the effects can continue for several hours or longer. Senna is available as an extract, or syrup, but most people prefer to take it in tablets to avoid its truly awful taste. The usual dosage is half a teaspoon for the liquid forms or one or two tablets. For a more mild laxative effect, try a cup of senna-leaf tea. Purchase senna-leaf tea bags at your health food store. Drink no more than one cup a day.

A South American herb called pau d'arco or lapacho also contains anthraquinones and is a useful mild laxative. The inner bark of the plant contains the active ingredients. You can purchase pau d'arco capsules at your health food store; start with one or two capsules and gradually increase the daily dose until you get results.

Cascara, buckthorn, senna, and pau d'arco should be avoided by pregnant women to avoid harming the fetus. Since the active ingredients can be passed on through breast milk, they should also be avoided by nursing women.

In traditional Chinese herbal medicine, rhubarb root, in powder or tincture form, is sometimes recommended as a laxative. Like senna and cascara, rhubarb root contains anthraquinones, which act as a powerful purgative. (The red rhubarb stalks found in the supermarket or grown in the garden have virtually no laxative effect.) Rhubarb root is generally quite potent and should be avoided, but the traditional Chinese herb *fo-ti* has a much more mild laxative effect.

Many traditional European or North American herbs, including yellow dock, dandelion root, and licorice root, are often recommended as stimulant laxatives, although we suggest you avoid them. Yellow dock has a laxative effect similar to rhubarb and should be avoided. Dandelion root does have a mild laxative effect, but it also acts as a diuretic (a substance that increases urine output) and should not be used. Licorice is basically worthless.

Aloe vera, in the form of juice or gel, is a very effective stimulant laxative. If you must use it, take no more than two ounces of the juice or two tablespoons of the gel once a day only until you get results. Aloe and rhubarb root are ingredients in a popular European herbal preparation called Swedish bitters. In small amounts Swedish bitters may be helpful for constipation, but avoid large doses and do not use it for more than a few days.

The castor bean, a popular ornamental plant, is the source of castor oil, a mild but foul-tasting laxative. The seeds that contain the oil also contain a dangerous chemical called ricin that can cause vomiting, diarrhea, blurred vision; small children can die from eating just a single seed. Don't use castor oil to treat constipation or anything else.

Vitamin and mineral supplements   Large doses of vitamin C have a mild laxative effect and can be useful as a stool softener. Too much vitamin C, however, can cause diarrhea. If you are constipated, try taking 1,000 to 2,000 milligrams of vitamin C. If that doesn't help within twenty-four hours, add another 500 milligrams to the dose. Taking 500 milligrams of vitamin C daily is a useful preventive measure if you often suffer from constipation.

Magnesium supplements have a more powerful laxative effect. Start with a low dose of no more than 400 milligrams and increase to no more than 1,000 milligrams as needed. Stop taking magnesium as soon as you move your bowels and do not use it on a regular basis—or you may risk chronic diarrhea.

Juice therapy   As mentioned above in the discussion of dietary treatments for constipation, prune juice contains a natural laxative called isatin. A daily six-ounce glass of prune juice will be very helpful for promoting regularity. Purchase bottled prune juice with no added sugar; this is readily available in any supermarket. Prune juice also contains sorbitol, however, which can cause diarrhea for some people. If you are sensitive to sorbitol, use prune juice cautiously in small amounts.

Fig juice is another well-known constipation remedy. You can purchase fig juice or fig juice concentrate in health food stores. Fig juice is extremely sweet, so we suggest diluting it with plain water or carrot juice, using one part fig juice and two parts of the other liquid. Fig juice concentrate needs to be diluted even further with at least three parts of other liquids. Start with one glass a day; you should get results within twenty-four hours. Do not use fig juice if you have diabetes or hypoglycemia.

Pure apple juice (no added water or sweeteners), or a mixture of equal amounts of pure apple and pear juice, is very helpful for relieving constipation, chiefly because of the large amounts of sorbitol in the juice. Especially if you are sensitive to sorbitol, start with eight ounces daily and increase to two cups daily until results occur. Do not use these juices if you have diabetes or hypoglycemia.

Some herbalists recommend a mixture of equal parts apple juice and spinach or parsley juice as a quick remedy for constipation. Start with eight ounces a day and increase to no more than two cups daily. You should experience results within forty-eight hours.

Fresh lemon juice can help stimulate the bowel and aid in evacuation. Combine the juice of half a lemon (about two tablespoons) with a cup of hot water and drink it first thing in the morning. Follow immediately with a glass of cold water or juice.

Hydrotherapy The importance of drinking enough water to prevent constipation has been discussed above, but we'd like to emphasize it again here. If you frequently are constipated, be sure to drink eight to twelve eight-ounce glasses of pure water every day. Many of our patients find that this is a cost-free and very effective cure. In addition to solving their constipation problem, getting the right amount of water also helps them feel better in general.

Homeopathy   A frequently recommended homeopathic remedy for constipation with dry, hard stools is natrum muriaticum 6x taken four times a day. Constipation with some gas or abdominal cramps may be relieved by graphites 6x taken four times a day. If you have large amounts of gas and are constipated, try lycopodium 6c every two hours for up to seven doses. Constipation that alternates with diarrhea is sometimes helped by nux vomica 6c taken four times a day. If you feel the urge to defecate but can't pass the stool, try nux vomica 6c every two hours; repeat up to ten doses.

Relaxation techniques   Sometimes constipation is alleviated by exercises that help relax the pelvic and abdominal muscles. In traditional yoga, the spine twist and the half shoulder stand are often suggested for constipation. Directions for these exercises can be found in any good book on yoga techniques.

Combined Treatments

Diet and hydrotherapy   To treat mild constipation and avoid it in the future, eat a high-fiber diet (at least thirty grams daily) and drink plenty of pure water (eight to twelve glasses daily).

Diet and juice therapy   If you are having a bout of constipation, increase the fiber in your diet and have an eight-ounce glass of prune juice in the morning. If this does not relieve your constipation within twenty-four

hours, increase the amount of prune juice to twelve
ounces.

Diet and natural laxatives   To deal with a bout of constipation, increase the fiber in your diet. Try using a mild
herbal stimulant laxative such as cascara, senna, or pau
d'arco. Start with a small dose and increase gradually
only if you have no results within twenty-four hours.
Stop using the laxative as soon as your constipation is
cleared up.

PARASITES

Parasites are tiny organisms that live within your intestinal tract, growing and feeding off your body and causing
only illness in return. The main symptoms of a parasite
infection are usually severe diarrhea and abdominal pain.
Other symptoms could include nausea, vomiting, gas and
bloating, foul-smelling stools, appetite and weight loss,
headache, constipation, blood or mucus in the stools, and
fatigue. In addition, digestive disruption or toxins created
by the parasite can cause muscle and joint pain, anemia,
allergies, chronic fatigue, and depression. If the parasites
aren't detected and treated quickly, the ongoing irritation
to your small intestine can cause leaky gut syndrome (see
chapter 6 for more information). Parasites can also compromise your immune system and make you more liable
to other serious health problems.

Harmful parasites are very common in the less developed world. Even in modern, sanitation-conscious America, a surprising number of people carry harmful parasites
such as *Giardia lamblia* and *Entamoeba hitolytica* in
their colon. You can get a parasitic infection by a number
of different transmission routes, although most involve

fecal contamination in some form. Raw or undercooked foods are one common transmission route; unsanitary restaurant practices are another. Lack of hygiene and unsanitary practices in other public places are another common route. *Giardia*, for example, is often spread among children through careless diaper changing and poor hygiene, especially in preschools and day care centers. *Giardia* can also be transmitted between sexual partners and in food and water. The main symptoms of giardiasis (infection with *Giardia*) are severe, foul-smelling diarrhea, gas, abdominal bloating, and nausea. Children with giardiasis have poor appetite, along with foul-smelling stools, listlessness, and weight loss.

As recent outbreaks have shown, *Cryptosporidium* can be spread through contaminated water supplies, including water that has been carefully treated at municipal treatment plants. The problem is that the chlorine added during treatment is not always enough to kill all the *Cryptosporidium* cysts. The major symptom of *Cryptosporidium* infection is severe, persistent diarrhea and cramps. Children and people with compromised immune systems can become very sick or even die from *Cryptosporidium* infection. If you suspect *Cryptosporidium* infection, get medical attention at once.

Helminths (worms) such as pinworms (also called threadworms) or roundworms can be transmitted by fecal contamination or through infected soil or water. The major symptom of pinworms is itching around the anus, especially at night. In the early stages of roundworm infection, there are few or no symptoms. When the roundworms have multiplied enough, they can cause stomach pain, nausea, and diarrhea.

Anyone can get a parasitic infection—you don't even

have to leave your house, much less travel to an exotic locale. If you have a health problem that isn't responding well to treatment, parasites could be the root cause. Treating the symptoms alone won't eliminate the parasites—the parasites themselves must be eliminated completely.

Although almost any persistent digestive problem could be caused by parasites, health care practitioners often don't test for their presence until they have run out of other ideas for diagnosing and treating the patient. Complicating the problem is the fact that parasites are sometimes hard to detect, even with standard lab tests. *Giardia*, for example, often goes undetected. All too often, patients end up being treated for the wrong problem. The best way to diagnose a parasite infection is through a comprehensive parasite test performed by a specialized laboratory. If your doctor recommends such a test, an ordinary stool sample will probably not be sufficient. Instead, you will have to provide a purged stool sample, which is usually produced by taking a saline laxative such as milk of magnesia. Your doctor will explain what and when to eat and when to take the laxative. It's important to follow the instructions carefully—you won't want to have to repeat the experience.

Traditional Treatments

Diet There is some evidence that a high-fiber diet can reduce the rate of parasitic infection, especially by *Giardia*. This may work because the fiber makes your colon produce more mucus and also speeds fecal transit time. These conditions make it harder for the parasites to establish themselves in your colon and begin reproducing; they are excreted instead.

Self-help steps   Prevention is by far the best way to prevent parasitic infections. Some simple, common-sense hygiene measures will help protect you and your family against parasites.

Avoid raw or undercooked foods, especially in restaurants; avoid restaurants that look unsanitary. At home, cook hamburger meat thoroughly (there should be no pink color left). Don't drink *any* untreated water, even if it comes from a "pure" mountain spring or looks clear. When traveling in less developed countries, drink only bottled or boiled water (see the section on diarrhea above for more sanitation advice for travelers). Always wash your hands thoroughly after any sort of contact with feces, human or animal. Insist on good hygiene and antiseptic cleaning practices at day care centers, schools, summer camps, and anyplace else your young children attend.

Because water-borne organisms such as *Cryptosporidium* are not always completely removed by your municipal water systems, I suggest installing an inexpensive water filtration device (Water Pure is an excellent choice) on your kitchen tap and drawing water for drinking and cooking only from that source. If your water is not treated at all (if it comes from your own well, for example), you should definitely install a good water filter. These filters remove most dangerous bacteria and parasites, and they also remove undesirable chemicals such as lead. If you prefer to use bottled water, purchase only pure filtered water in glass containers.

If you have been infected with intestinal worms, careful attention to hygiene is important to prevent reinfection. All members of your household should wash their hands frequently, particularly after bowel movements and before meals. All bathrooms should be thoroughly disinfected. Pinworm eggs can get into bedding, nightclothes, underwear, and other clothing, and they can then cause reinfection later. Wash all bedding and clothing soon after you take the medication your doctor suggests. Vacuum all carpets and rugs, especially those near beds.

Parasites can be transmitted through fresh produce, which may have been handled in an unsanitary manner during harvesting or shipping. Always wash fresh fruits and vegetables before using them. The best way to do this is to mix two tablespoons of distilled vinegar in a gallon of filtered tap water. Soak the produce for fifteen minutes, then drain, rinse, and dry.

Drugs Antiparasitic drugs (also called antiprotozoal drugs) and anti-worm drugs (also called anthelmintic drugs) are fairly powerful but also very effective. If you need to take one of these drugs, your doctor will discuss possible side effects with you; in general, these are not severe. You will probably have to take the drug for ten to twenty days; the side effects stop when you stop taking the drug. It is very important to have a repeat stool test a month after you finish the medication to make sure all the parasites have been eliminated.

For infection with an amoeba such as *Entamoeba histolytica*, doctors usually prescribe iodoquinol (Diquinol, Yodoxin, or the generic equivalent) or paromomycin (Humatin) if you have no symptoms. In rare cases, iodoquinol may cause blurred vision; it also sometimes causes a rash, acne, nausea, or abdominal cramps. If you do have symptoms from parasites, your doctor will probably prescribe metronidazole (Flagyl, Metizol, or the generic equivalent). Do not drink alcohol or take any alcohol-based medicines if you are taking metronidazole.

Metronidazole can sometimes cause nausea, headache, or dry mouth; it may also cause a temporary, harmless darkening of the urine.

If you have giardiasis, your doctor will probably prescribe metronidazole or possibly quinacrine (Atabrine). Take this drug after meals with a full glass of liquid. A common side effect of quinacrine is a harmless, temporary yellow discoloration of the skin and urine. The yellow color goes away when you stop taking the drug. A less common side effect of quinacrine is dizziness. If you are infected with *Blastocystis hominis*, a common parasite that often causes no symptoms at all, your doctor will probably prescribe a medicine only if you develop symptoms. If you do, metronidazole or iodoquinol will probably be prescribed. Another effective medicine for giardiasis is tinidazole.

Infection with intestinal worms such as pinworms (enterobiasis) or roundworms (ascariasis), is fairly common, especially among young children. The original infection is usually acquired through unsanitary conditions; it is then easily passed among family members. Detecting pinworms is quite simple: a piece of clear cellophane tape is pressed against the anus and removed; if the worms are present, some will stick to the tape and be clearly visible.

Pinworms are very easy to transmit from person to person. Everyone in your household may need treatment at the same time to prevent reinfection. In addition, your whole family may need to be treated again in two to three weeks to clear up the worms completely. Your doctor will probably suggest an over-the-counter anthelmintic drug containing pyrantel (Antiminth, Reese's Pinworm Medication, or the generic equivalent). This drug works by paralyzing the worms, which are then passed from your body with your stool. You generally need to take just one dose in the form of a pleasant-tasting liquid. Once you've taken the drug, the worms will pass naturally—there's no need for any sort of laxative or enema.

Alternative Treatments

Herbal therapy   A number of herbs are commonly recommended for treating parasites, especially intestinal worms. Herbal remedies are often effective, but they take a long time to do the job—you will probably need to take the herb every day for at least a month. In the meantime, your symptoms will persist. In addition, unless you completely eliminate the parasites, they will return. Continue to take the remedy even after your symptoms improve. Use the herbal remedies discussed below only if you have a very mild infection.

Goldenseal, which contains an alkaloid called berberine sulfate, can help kill off parasites, particularly intestinal worms and *Giardia*. To make an infusion of goldenseal, steep two teaspoons of dried goldenseal root in one cup of boiling water for fifteen minutes. Strain before drinking and take no more than three cups a day. If you prefer capsules, try 500 to 1,000 milligrams of the freeze-dried root three times a day. In liquid form, use one to two teaspoons of the tincture or half a teaspoon of the fluid extract three times a day. Many people mix the fluid into a glass of water or fruit juice. Continue the treatment daily for one month.

Garlic is a traditional herbal remedy for intestinal worms, especially pinworms. The allicin in the garlic is also helpful for giardiasis. Many herbalists suggest eating one large raw garlic clove daily for three to four weeks. Some people like to chop the garlic and mix it with honey. Others prefer the simpler method of taking odor-less garlic capsules or tablets, available at any drugstore or health food store from a number of different manufac-turers. Eating a small raw onion every day may also help kill off worms. As with garlic, the onion may be chopped and mixed with honey. Do not, however, use dried or de-hydrated onions. Continue for three weeks to four weeks.

Grapefruit seed extract is said to help expel intestinal worms. Take up to 1,000 milligrams a day with food for three to four weeks.

Pumpkin seeds are a traditional Native American rem-edy for intestinal worms. The seeds contain oils that have anthelmintic properties. If you want to try this, purchase unsalted roasted pumpkin seeds at a health food store. Eat half a cup a day for two weeks; chew the seeds thor-oughly. Pumpkin seed is also available in extract form at well-stocked health food stores. Follow the instructions on the label.

Black walnut extract, a very bitter substance high in natural tannins, is a traditional folk remedy for intestinal worms. It is available at well-stocked health food stores; follow the instructions on the label.

In traditional Chinese herbal medicine, wormwood (also called artemisia annua) is suggested for intestinal worms. Since this herb has a very bitter taste, capsules or tablets are preferred; take one or two a day for a week; re-peat again for a week two weeks later. To make an infu-sion, steep two teaspoons of the dried herb in one cup of boiling water for fifteen minutes; strain before drinking. To kill worms most effectively, drink half a cup daily for a week in small amounts spread throughout the day. Re-peat again for a week two weeks later.

Vitamin and mineral supplements While you are suffering from a parasitic infection, your digestion is impaired and you may not be absorbing enough vitamins and minerals from your food. You also need extra nutrients to ward off secondary infections. On a daily basis take 2,000 milligrams of vitamin C, 25,000 IU of mixed carotenes, 25 milligrams of a complete B complex supplement, and 20 milligrams of zinc. In addition, take your usual multivitamin and mineral supplement.

Juice therapy Juices that contain the strong-smelling sulfur compounds in onions and garlic are helpful for killing intestinal worms. Most herbalists suggest a ratio of one teaspoon of liquid garlic (Kyolic is an excellent brand available in any drugstore) per quarter cup of fresh onion juice. Combine this with as much fresh carrot or other vegetable juice as you need to make the mixture palatable. Drink enough of the mixture to get a quarter cup of onion juice in the morning on an empty stomach; repeat the dose at night before going to sleep. Continue for a week. Repeat again for a week two weeks later.

In traditional Chinese herbal medicine, persimmon juice is used to treat intestinal worms. Unripe persimmons are very high in tannins, which help paralyze the worms and thus make it easier to expel them with the feces. Unfortunately, unripe persimmons are very, very bitter to the taste. To make the juice, purchase fresh persimmons and let them start ripening at room temperature for several days. The fruits will be ready when they're soft enough to juice; the taste will still be quite bitter. Peel the fruits and juice the pulp. To make it palatable, mix the persimmon juice with an equal amount of apple juice. Drink half a cup in the morning on an empty stomach and another half cup at night before going to sleep. Continue for a week. Repeat again for a week two weeks later.

In traditional Ayurvedic medicine, pomegranate juice is used to treat intestinal worms. The bitter-tasting tannins in the juice kill or paralyze the worms and let them be eliminated. Pomegranate juice is difficult to make at home. Instead, purchase the unsweetened juice at your health food store. If you can't find the unsweetened kind, cut the juice with equal amounts of water; the added sugar could cause diarrhea, especially in children. Drink half a cup in the morning on an empty stomach and another half cup at night before going to sleep. Continue for a week. Repeat again for a week two weeks later.

Homeopathic remedies   Homeopaths usually suggest treating pinworms with Cina 6c (also called artemisia or wormseed) taken three times daily for two weeks or Teucrium 6c taken three times daily for two weeks. Some homeopaths also suggest sabadilla 6c taken three times daily for two weeks.

Caution   Do not follow the old folk remedy of drinking turpentine or kerosene for intestinal worms! Do not use high colonics, enemas, saline laxatives, castor oil, or anything else to "purge" the intestines of worms.

Combined Treatments

Medication and prevention   Most parasitic infections respond very well to standard medicines. Prevention through good sanitation is the best cure, however.

Garlic and prevention   Mild cases of pinworm sometimes clear up when treated with garlic. Careful attention to hygiene is needed to keep the infection from spreading to other household members and to avoid reinfection.

CHAPTER 9

Other Problems of the Large Intestine

As we've already discussed in the previous chapter, relatively minor and self-limiting colon problems such as flatulence, diarrhea, and constipation are quite common. Numerous more serious health problems can also arise in the colon. In this chapter, we'll start with a discussion of the toxic bowel and its possible health consequences. We'll also discuss the causes and treatments of ailments such as irritable bowel syndrome, Crohn's disease, appendicitis, and cancer of the colon.

Your colon contains literally trillions of bacteria from some four hundred different species. In the healthy bowel, most of these bacteria are beneficial—in fact, they are vital. One of their major functions is to ferment ingested material and convert it into short-chain fatty acids such as butyric acid (also called butyrate) and acetic acid. Butyric acid is the primary fuel for nourishing and repairing the cells that line the colon; it also inhibits the growth of cancerous cells in the colon. Acetic acid may help lower blood cholesterol levels by affecting your liver, where most of your cholesterol is produced.

Lactobacilli, including the friendly bacteria *Lacto-*

bacillus acidophilus and *Lactobacillus bifidus*, are the most abundant and most important of your bowel bacteria. These bacteria produce natural antibiotics that help kill dangerous pathogens such as salmonella, *E. coli*, and staphylococcus. They also inhibit the growth of the unfriendly, yeastlike organism *Candida albicans*. Among many other functions, lactobacilli also synthesize B vitamins and vitamin K, reduce flatulence, and remove environmental toxins from your body.

Good bowel function and a healthy colon are at the heart of much modern thinking in alternative medicine. And at the heart of good bowel function is sufficient dietary fiber, for without enough fiber, the beneficial bacteria starve. But what is fiber and why is it so important?

In the 1970s, two British doctors, Denis Burkitt and Hugh Trowell, were studying disease in Uganda. They realized that their patients suffered from very few of the ailments closely associated with Western lifestyles. In particular, their African patients only rarely suffered from bowel problems such as constipation, diverticulitis, colon cancer, and hemorrhoids. They had a low incidence of metabolic problems such as diabetes, obesity, and gallstones, and they also had a low incidence of heart disease, stroke, high blood pressure, and varicose veins. Noting that their patients ate primarily unprocessed foods that were very high in dietary fiber, which caused them to have large and frequent bowel movements, the doctors concluded that a high-fiber diet can help prevent certain illnesses, especially those digestive illnesses closely associated with the typical low-fiber, high-fat Western diet.

Dietary fiber consists of the indigestible parts of plant foods. These fall into two basic categories: insoluble fiber and soluble fiber. Consisting primarily of cellulose (which forms the walls of plant cells), insoluble fiber has the ability to absorb water in the intestines. This makes the fiber swell up, forming a large, bulky stool that is easily passed from the body. Good sources of insoluble fiber include wheat bran, whole grains, beans and peas, and the skins of fruits and vegetables.

Soluble fiber consists primarily of pectin, along with mucilage, plant gums, and hemicellulose. Because soluble fiber dissolves in water, it forms a gel as it moves through your intestines. The gel slows the absorption of some nutrients from the intestine into the bloodstream and also adds to the bulk and softness of the stool. Good dietary sources of soluble fiber include oat bran, beans, fruit, and some vegetables.

By making your stool large, soft, and easy to eliminate, fiber reduces straining during bowel movements. This in turn reduces the likelihood of diverticulosis, diverticulitis, hemorrhoids, and varicose veins. By slowing the absorption of nutrients into your system, fiber can help keep your blood sugar levels steady—a boon to diabetics. Soluble fiber can help lower your blood cholesterol levels by binding bile acids and increasing the elimination of cholesterol in the feces. A diet high in fiber could lower your risk of polyps and cancer of the colon. And as we've discussed, fiber also nourishes the trillions of beneficial bacteria found in your colon and nourishes the colon itself.

THE TOXIC BOWEL

If you don't get enough dietary fiber, your body's waste products remain in the colon longer than they should. If this happens only occasionally, you might have temporary constipation, gas, bloating, or diarrhea, problems that go away when you add more fiber to your diet. If you routinely eat a low-fiber diet, however, you could starve and weaken the desirable bacteria in your colon and let the unfriendly bacteria get the upper hand. In general, too low a level of friendly bacteria in your bowel means you will have markedly lower resistance to gastrointestinal illnesses, especially those that cause diarrhea. More significantly, you could also have more severe health problems caused by putrefaction or fermentation excess.

If your diet is high in fats and animal protein and low in fiber, your stool will move slowly through your colon. A deficiency of fiber means a deficiency of friendly bacteria and thus of short-chain fatty acids for nourishing the colon. The combination of too little fiber and too much fat gives the various unfriendly *Bacteroides* bacteria in your bowel plenty of their favorite food, however, and they will produce plenty of urease as a waste product. Your kidneys and liver will have to work overtime to remove the urease from your system. In addition, conditions will be right for the anaerobic bacteria in your bowel to flourish, causing an unfavorable decrease in the number of aerobic (oxygen-breathing) bacteria. The anaerobic bacteria may cause a decrease in the amount of butyric acid available to nourish the cells of the colon. They may also digest bile acids in the feces and convert them into byproducts that encourage tumor formation.

When organisms such as *Candida albicans* have no natural check in your bowel, they can multiply with amazing rapidity, causing an overgrowth that leads to excess bacterial fermentation. The usual symptoms include bloating, gas, diarrhea alternating with constipation, and feelings of malaise or fatigue. In more severe cases, toxins released by the yeastlike *Candida* and by bacteria may enter your blood and circulate in your body, causing fatigue, muscle and joint pain, depression, mood swings, and autoimmune diseases. In addition, the circulating bowel toxins put an extra strain on your liver and may cause many other unpleasant symptoms, including bad breath, nausea, headaches, boils, eczema, and possibly food allergies. The infection could also spread to other parts of your body, including the vagina (yeast infection) and the mouth (oral thrush). Another possible consequence of bacterial overgrowth is too many unfriendly *Clostridium* bacteria in your colon. *Clostridium* produce a toxin from the bile acids in your stool that is related to colon cancer.

Although too little dietary fiber is usually the cause of bowel toxicity, other factors can also trigger the problem. Drugs such as antibiotics, steroids, and birth control pills can throw off the balance of good and bad bacteria. Too much sugar in the diet is another possible trigger. If you eat too little fiber, too much sugar, *and* take an antibiotic, you are even more likely to have a problem.

Because the symptoms of a toxic bowel are sometimes vague or changeable, traditional physicians may not notice them or may suggest they are "psychological." In fact, toxic bowel is a fairly straightforward diagnosis. A history of infrequent bowel movements (fewer than one a day) or of constipation is a good clue; so is a history of alternating constipation and diarrhea. Another important step in arriving at a diagnosis is to measure bowel transit time, as discussed in chapter 8. If the transit time is more than twenty-four hours, toxic bowel should be suspected. A urinary indican test (also sometimes called an Obermeyer test) can be used to measure how much indican is in the urine. Since indican is a byproduct made when the beneficial bacteria in your bowel digest the amino acids phenylalanine, tryptophan, and tyrosine, the amount present in your urine provides a useful indication of bowel function. If your bowel transit time is slow, the bacteria have more time to ferment the bowel contents; the longer the fermentation goes on, the more indican enters your blood and is excreted in your urine, and the higher your level will be when your urine is tested. Similarly, you will have a high indican level if you have a lot of unfriendly bacteria, even if your transit time is good.

An excellent method for diagnosing toxic bowel and assessing the extent of the problem is the comprehensive digestive stool analysis (CDSA), which evaluates metabolic markers and bacteria in your colon and provides a good picture of your bowel's state of health. If you wish to have a CDSA performed, discuss it with your health care provider. It's important to choose a reliable laboratory that can do complete and accurate testing.

Several metabolic markers in the stool provide good indications of overall colon health. The pH, or acidity, of the stool is one such indicator. The normal pH range is 6 to 7.2. An alkaline pH (above 7) may indicate a shortage of butyric acid, which in turn could mean that your colon is not getting adequate nourishment. Too much acid in the stool could be an indication that you need more fiber in your diet. Analyzing the short-chain fatty acids (SCFAs) in the stool also provides valuable information. SCFAs such as acetate, propionate, butyrate, and valerate are produced by the bacteria in the colon when they ferment soluble fiber. These acids are vital for nourishing the colon: SCFAs provide up to 70 percent of the energy for the cells that line the colon, for example. They are also important for maintaining colon health and for keeping harmful bacteria such as salmonella and shigella from establishing themselves in the colon and causing illness. If your SCFAs are elevated, you may have a bacterial overgrowth or colitis. If your SCFAs are too low, that too could indicate a bacterial overgrowth or too little soluble fiber in the diet. Similarly, if your SCFAs are out of balance, with a higher proportion of one or two SCFAs compared to the others, you could have a bacterial overgrowth or intestinal infection. The CDSA also looks at your levels of butyric acid. Since butyrate, the most important SCFA, is produced from butyric acid you need to have adequate amounts. A persistent shortage of butyric acid could be related to colitis, inflammatory bowel disease, or even colon cancer.

Another important metabolic marker is the level of beta-glucuronidase in the stool. The substance is an enzyme produced by some unfriendly bacteria in the bowel. It may break down other substances produced by the same bacteria in the bowel and cause them to become carcinogenic. Excess beta-glucuronidase may be correlated with increased cancer risk, particularly estrogen-related cancers such as breast cancer. Because beta-glucuronidase affects estrogen, high levels of it may also be responsible for some cases of premenstrual stress. Low levels may indicate dysbiosis, particularly dysbiosis from antoboitic treatment.

The comprehensive digestive stool analysis also studies the bacteria—both friendly and unfriendly—in the stool. An imbalance in the bacteria could indicate a bacterial overgrowth problem.

Traditional Treatments

Diet   Increasing the amount of fiber in your diet and eliminating junk foods, highly processed foods, and excessive sugar are important steps for restoring good bowel function and a proper balance of beneficial bacteria. Adding fiber provides fuel for the beneficial bacteria so that they can produce adequate amounts of butyric acid for colon nourishment. In addition, fiber helps your stool move through your colon quickly and easily, so that undesirable bacteria and the toxins they release are eliminated efficiently.

The average American adult eats only about ten grams of dietary fiber a day. For good bowel function, most health care providers today suggest that you ingest at least twenty grams, and preferably thirty grams, a day. The best, simplest, and healthiest way to add fiber to your diet is by slowly increasing the amount of fresh or lightly cooked fruits and vegetables, whole grain foods, and beans you eat. You can easily get twenty grams of fiber a day by eating two to three servings of fruit, three servings of whole grains, and three or four servings of vegetables. The portions don't need to be large. One medium apple has about three grams of fiber, almost all water-soluble pectin. A cup of broccoli has about six grams of insoluble fiber. Breakfast cereals such as All-Bran have over eight grams of fiber per serving. Because fiber-rich foods are also filling and satisfying, many patients easily lose some weight when they start eating more fiber.

As you start adding more fiber to your diet, it's important to do it slowly and by eating a variety of fiber-rich food. If you become gassy or bloated, eat less fiber until the symptoms disappear, then slowly include additional fiber. Be sure to drink plenty of fluids—six to eight eight-ounce glasses a day or even more—as you eat more fiber.

Eliminating or sharply reducing the amounts of processed foods and sugar you eat will also help restore a good balance of bacteria to your colon by taking away the foods that unfriendly bacteria most like to digest.

Fermented foods are often very helpful for restoring a good balance of friendly bacteria in the bowel. In mild cases of bacterial overgrowth that do not involve *Candida albicans* (a yeastlike organism), adding fermented dairy products such as unflavored live-culture yogurt can help by restoring some favorable bacteria to your small intestine. Most supermarket yogurt does not contain live cultures, so you'll probably have to purchase live-culture yogurt at your health food store. Try having several ounces just before each meal.

Self-help steps   Having regular, full bowel movements is vital for preventing toxic bowel problems. Eating plenty of fiber, drinking enough fluids (eight eight-ounce glasses a day), and exercising gently every day is the best way to ensure regularity. (For more information, see the section on constipation in chapter 8.) Although some health care practitioners recommend enemas or colonic irrigation for severe cases of bowel toxicity, we feel this is not needed and could do more harm than good, since these methods remove both good and bad bacteria and do not deal with the underlying causes of the problem. They can also lead to dangerous electrolyte imbalances. Discuss enemas and colonic irrigation with your health care provider before you try them.

Drugs   In severe cases of bacterial overgrowth or *Candida* infections, broad-spectrum antibiotics such as amoxicillin or metronidazole (Flagyl) are often helpful.

Prescription antibiotic drugs such as penicillin or tetracycline kill off all aerobic bacteria, both good and bad, in your intestines. The shortage of aerobic bacteria can allow undesirable anaerobic bacteria or *Candida albicans* to take over in your large and small intestines, particularly if you must take the antibiotic for a long time. If your doctor prescribes these drugs, it is usually because you need them for an infection or illness. However, sometimes antibiotics are routinely prescribed for colds or flu, which are viral illnesses that are not helped by antibiotics. Discuss the necessity for antibiotics with your doctor. If you must take the drug, we strongly suggest that you also eat some plain, live-culture yogurt every day. Since most antibiotics work best when taken on an empty stomach, and because dairy products in particular can interfere with their action, it's best to eat several ounces of the yogurt two to three hours after taking each pill.

Alternative Treatments

Beneficial bacteria supplements   Many patients are able to restore a good balance of beneficial bacteria to the colon by taking bacteria supplements along with nutrients that help the bacteria reestablish themselves. The beneficial bacteria multiply in the small intestine and colon with the help of the nutrients and crowd out the bad bacteria and yeast.

Supplements of high-quality acidophilus, bulgaricus, bifidobacteria, or lactobacillus in powder form help add back beneficial bacteria. A type of yeast called *Saccharomyces boulardii* is also helpful for normalizing the bowel bacteria and creating a good environment for friendly bacteria. Many different beneficial bacteria supplements are available. To select a good product, look for those that contain only one type of bacteria, preferably the DDS-1 acidophilus strain or the *Malyoth bifidobacteria* strain. The product should be cultured in a milk-based medium and then ultrafiltered, not centrifuged. Finally, the product should be certified to contain at least one billion active bacteria per gram. Purchase the supplement only if you know it has been kept refrigerated and does not contain the bacteria *Lactobacillus casei* or *Streptococcus faecium*.

To get the maximum benefit from friendly bacteria supplements, combine acidophilus and bifidobacteria supplements with *S. boulardii*. The usual daily dosage for a mild bacterial overgrowth problem is one gram (about half a level teaspoon) of acidophilus with 250 milligrams (about an eighth of a teaspoon) of bifidobacteria. Mix the powders in three ounces of pure, chlorine-free cold water and drink the mixture on an empty stomach about ten to fifteen minutes before eating. If you prefer, take the bacteria in capsules with a full glass of pure water. In addition, take one or two 300-milligram capsules of *S. boulardii* on the same schedule.

Taking the bacteria on an empty stomach seems to help them survive the powerful acids of your stomach and arrive safely in the ileum (or lower portion of your small intestine). From there, the bacteria will be naturally moved on to the colon along with the feces.

If you have a serious bacterial overgrowth or if your overgrowth is affecting your liver function, you may need to take between five and ten grams of acidophilus and up to six grams of bifidobacteria daily, spread out between meals during the day; take two 300-milligram capsules of *S. boulardii* with each dose. In addition, you may wish to add supplements of *Lactobacillus bulgarica*. This bacteria is most effective when three to six grams are taken with meals.

Once the bacteria arrive in the lower part of your small intestine, they need some nutritional help to regain their foothold. Most practitioners recommend taking fructooligosaccharides (FOS) along with your beneficial bacteria supplements. Supplements of FOS fuel the growth of beneficial bacteria in the gut. Because they are not broken down and digested by your body, they are completely available only to the bacteria. Low levels of FOS are found naturally in some foods such as honey and garlic; artichoke flour contains higher levels of FOS. To get the real benefits of FOS, however, the higher concentrations of 95 percent pure powder or syrup are most helpful. Since FOS products are mildly sweet, they can be used as a sweetener in beverages or on food, although they don't work very well as a sugar substitute in cooking. Alternatively, you can swallow them as tablets. Start with one gram (about a quarter teaspoon) a day and gradually increase the dose to three or four grams daily. Large amounts of FOS can cause mild diarrhea in some people. If this occurs, reduce your daily dose until you return to normal.

After the bacteria are reestablished in the small intestine, they will be naturally moved on into the colon. Soluble fiber is needed to fuel the growth of the bacteria in your colon. In addition to taking the bacteria supplements and FOS, then, you will need to add soluble fiber to your diet. Eat at least one piece of fresh, organically grown fruit, which includes peaches, apples, bananas, or pears, with each meal. Gradually add more fiber to your diet by eating more fresh vegetables and whole grains.

When you first start to take beneficial bacteria for problems of the large intestine, you may have a temporary worsening of symptoms, including gas and diarrhea, as the bad bacteria die off suddenly and release toxins. Although this is perfectly normal, you can avoid the discomfort by starting with small doses and gradually increasing them. Cut back on the dosage if your symptoms become too unpleasant.

Other supplements   Whey tablets (made from the watery part of milk left over when the curds are removed to make cheese) help nourish and restore the friendly bacteria in the bowel. Take one tablet along with each dose of beneficial bacteria. Whey may cause flatulence and other problems if you are lactose intolerant or allergic to milk.

Herbal therapy   If constipation is a problem for you, try gentle herbal remedies such as flaxseed (see the section on constipation in chapter 8 for more information).

Juice therapy   Fresh lemon juice can help stimulate the bowel and aid in evacuation. Combine the juice of half a lemon (about two tablespoons) with a cup of hot water and drink it first thing in the morning. Green juices that contain chlorophyll are also helpful for the bowel. Try having eight ounces daily of fresh green juice made from wheatgrass, alfalfa, spinach, parsley, or any green leafy vegetable, singly or in combination.

Combined Treatments

Diet and beneficial bacteria supplements   Bowel toxicity almost always results from too little fiber in the diet. Adding fiber through the foods you eat will help the problem quite a bit. At the same time, taking beneficial bacteria supplements will help beneficial bacteria reestablish themselves in your colon.

IRRITABLE BOWEL SYNDROME

Crampy pain, gassiness, bloating, diarrhea, constipation, mucus in the stool, and changes in bowel habits are often signs of irritable bowel syndrome (IBS), an ailment that affects at least 10 to 15 percent of all American adults. IBS is actually second only to the common cold as a cause of missed workdays. Irritable bowel syndrome can be severe and cause a great deal of distress and discomfort, especially if all the symptoms are present or if you have frequent bouts. Many people with IBS, however, have only one or two of the symptoms when they have occasional attacks. You are most likely to develop the symptoms of IBS as a young adult—in your late teens or early twenties; young women are much more likely to have it than young men. If you have IBS, you are likely to have it for life, although it will probably not get any worse than when it first starts and it may go away for long periods or even forever. In most cases, IBS is not a serious medical problem and it does not lead to any serious diseases such as cancer. You can do a lot to help yourself if you have IBS, since it responds very well to diet and other treatments.

In the past, IBS was often called functional bowel disease, colitis, mucus colitis, or spastic colon, but these terms are no longer used. IBS should not be confused with ulcerative colitis or inflammatory bowel diseases such as colitis.

Irritable bowel syndrome can be hard to diagnose. Someone who experiences gas and diarrhea once every few months, for example, might just attribute the problem to a stomach virus and never realize that IBS is the real culprit. There is no diagnostic test for IBS. In fact, a diagnosis of IBS is generally confirmed when the colon appears normal, there is no intestinal bleeding, and all the usual medical tests come back normal. When all other possible causes of the symptoms have been eliminated and yet the symptoms persist, IBS is almost certainly the problem.

Although stress can bring on or worsen IBS symptoms, IBS has a physical origin, not a psychosomatic one. The symptoms occur because your colon doesn't contract properly. It may contract too forcefully, causing cramps and diarrhea, or it may not contract enough, causing constipation. Often the bowel alternates between the two extremes, causing alternating bouts of diarrhea and constipation. Why doesn't your colon contract as it should? Researchers are still investigating that question. One theory is that someone with IBS has a colon that is more sensitive and reactive than usual, so it responds more strongly to stimuli that wouldn't bother most people. For example, the ordinary act of eating, which has no effect on most people, could trigger an overreaction in someone with IBS. Stress worsens the symptoms because the colon is controlled in part by your nervous system. Hormonal changes may also play a role. Many women find that their IBS symptoms are worse when they are menstruating.

In some cases, IBS patients have unsuspected intestinal parasites. If you have IBS, talk to your doctor about having a comprehensive digestive stool analysis to find any hidden parasites (see chapter 8 for more information about detecting and treating parasites).

Every patient with IBS is different, with different symptoms, different flare-up triggers, and different responses to treatment. If you have IBS, work with your health care provider to develop a treatment plan that works well for you. You may also find that meeting with fellow IBS sufferers in a support group is very helpful. To find a support group near you, contact:

International Foundation for Bowel Dysfunction
Box 17864
Milwaukee, WI 53217
(414) 964-1799

Traditional Treatments

Diet   A two-pronged approach to diet is crucial for controlling your IBS symptoms. Adding fiber to the diet is one prong of the approach; the other is discovering the foods that trigger your symptoms.

In many cases, additional dietary fiber will help control the symptoms of irritable bowel syndrome. High-fiber foods such as bran, whole grains, beans, fruits, and vegetables help prevent constipation and normalize watery bowel movements. Many doctors also suggest taking over-the-counter fiber supplements containing psyllium husks. Add fiber to your diet gradually and carefully. Too much raw food, for example, could make your symptoms worse. Try eating steamed vegetables and stewed fruits; avoid beans, cabbage, and other gas-producing foods if gas is a problem. Even so, at first you may experience some bloating, gas, and other symptoms. As your system gets used to the additional fiber, this should diminish, but the overall benefits of adding fiber may take a few weeks or even a few months to be apparent. Be sure to drink six to eight eight-ounce glasses of liquid every day as well—fiber needs to absorb water to help.

Many people with IBS have specific food sensitivities that are individual to them. By identifying the problem foods and avoiding them, they can often sharply reduce or even eliminate their symptoms. A good way to do this is to keep a food diary for a few weeks. Note what you eat at each meal and in between; also note your symptoms. You should soon be able to relate specific foods to specific reactions. Since every IBS patient has different food sensitivities, only you can determine which foods are triggers for you.

Lactose intolerance (the inability to digest milk products) is quite common among IBS sufferers. The best treatment is to avoid lactose in all forms. (See the discussion of lactose intolerance in chapter 5 for more information on this problem.)

Fatty foods are another very common IBS trigger, often causing colon contractions that lead to painful spasms or diarrhea. Eating a low-fat diet in general is often helpful. Specifically, avoid fried foods, red meat, luncheon meats, and high-fat snack foods.

Caffeine from coffee, tea, and soft drinks can also trigger colon contractions. Cut back on caffeine or avoid it completely. Spicy foods can also trigger problems, although this varies widely from person to person.

Corn, wheat, the food additive monosodium glutamate (MSG), artificial sweeteners such as sorbitol, and other food additives such as nitrates and nitrites are other common IBS triggers. Avoid these foods and any others that you know aggravate your IBS symptoms.

Sugar of any sort, including sucrose, fructose, glucose, corn syrup, and the others, often makes IBS worse, causing diarrhea, gas, and bloating. Many IBS patients find that a completely sugar-free diet relieves their symptoms quite a bit. This means avoiding fruits, fruit juice, candies, cookies, pastries, chocolate, and many other foods. In addition, many prepared foods such as salad dressings contain hidden sugar. Read all food labels very carefully.

Alcohol, carbonated beverages, and chewing gum can all worsen IBS symptoms.

If you have an IBS flare-up, treat your digestive system gently. Avoid the foods discussed above and any other foods that you know cause problems for you. Until your symptoms subside, eat easily digested foods such as rice, steamed vegetables, oatmeal, baked potatoes, steamed or baked white fish, and the like. Once you're feeling better, gradually return to your normal diet by adding one more food every day or two.

Many people with IBS have symptoms following or even during a meal. The larger the meal or the more fat it contains, the worse the symptoms may be. Eating fast-food meals or "eating on the run" can also trigger symptoms. One way to keep meals from triggering IBS symptoms is to eat smaller portions or to eat smaller meals more often. Try to eat regular, unhurried meals in pleasant surroundings; eat slowly and chew your food thoroughly.

Self-help steps   Stress and anxiety make your IBS symptoms worse, although they are not the cause of IBS. If you are in a troubled relationship, unhappy with your job, or have some other major stresses in your life, your IBS will probably be worse, and the symptoms may improve or even go away completely once the problems are resolved. The most important thing, however, is simply to acknowledge that stress does make your IBS worse. Professional counseling often helps IBS patients—especially those who have been newly diagnosed—learn to recognize and cope with stresses that trigger their bowel symptoms.

Your lifestyle has an effect on IBS. Overwork, too little sleep or irregular sleep patterns, smoking, alcohol, and recreational drugs can all worsen your symptoms.

Regular moderate exercise has a very positive effect on

IBS. Even going for a short walk every day can help. Low-impact aerobics, swimming, walking, bike riding, and the like are all helpful.

Uncomfortable abdominal cramps can often be relieved with a hot-water bottle or heating pad.

Drugs The painful cramps of IBS can be relieved with prescription antispasmodic drugs containing belladonna and barbiturates (Donnatal or the generic equivalent) or dicyclomine (Bentyl or the generic equivalent). These drugs should be used only to relieve an attack; they should not be taken on a regular basis. Side effects of these drugs can include dry mouth, dizziness, and blurred vision.

For some people with IBS, diarrhea is the most common symptom. Your doctor may recommend a nonprescription antidiarrheal medicine containing loperamide (Imodium or the generic equivalent) to help relieve the symptoms. If your diarrhea alternates with constipation, however, this could make the constipation worse.

Nonprescription antidiarrheal medications such as loperamide can be very useful for avoiding crises and letting you enjoy a normal lifestyle. For example, if you will be going somewhere that has no bathroom facilities (a long bus ride, perhaps), take your antidiarrheal medication before leaving home.

Constipation alternating with diarrhea is another common IBS symptom. If you are constipated, treat the problem with added fiber and liquid in your diet. Do not use any sort of laxative—this will make the later diarrhea phase more severe.

Antacids that contain magnesium may trigger diarrhea in people with IBS. Discuss the use of antacids with your health care provider.

Surgery   Surgery is not used as a treatment for irritable bowel syndrome.

Alternative Treatments

Acupressure/acupuncture   Acupressure techniques for relieving constipation are often helpful for IBS. For mild constipation, apply pressure to a point on your abdomen halfway between your navel and pubic bone. Lie flat on your back on a firm surface and place the fingertips of one hand on the point. Press down firmly and hold for thirty seconds. Repeat five more times.

A trained acupuncturist will discuss your IBS symptoms with you and then use techniques that both deal with specific problems of constipation or diarrhea and also generally relax your body.

Reflexology   Mild constipation from IBS can be helped by massaging the large intestine points on the soles of your feet and the palms of your hands. These points are located between the arch and the heel, on the inner side of each foot. There are several different points that correspond to the ascending, transverse, descending, and sigmoid colons, but applying steady pressure to the overall area is generally sufficient to provide relief. Two points on each palm correspond to the colon. The first point is about an inch below your fourth finger. The second point, which corresponds more closely with the sigmoid colon, is just above your wrist in line with your third finger. Apply steady pressure by rotating your thumb or a golf ball on the hand points. Repeat as needed.

Massaging the liver point on the top of each foot may also help constipation, especially if you feel bloated or "clogged." This point is found between the big and second toes just below the bottom joint.

Chiropractic treatments Chiropractic adjustment can sometimes relieve IBS symptoms, especially constipation. Chiropractic treatment is also often useful for relieving stress in general.

Herbal therapy Herbal remedies that add fiber naturally are a good way to help control IBS symptoms. Unsweetened breakfast cereals that contain large amounts of bran (the fibrous outer coating of grains such as wheat, oats, corn, or rice) are a good approach—but avoid any that cause symptoms for you, as may be the case with wheat or corn. If you prefer, purchase pure bran and sprinkle a few teaspoons on your regular breakfast cereal. As a bonus, bran, especially rice bran and oat bran, may help reduce your blood cholesterol levels.

Psyllium, the ingredient found in many bulk-forming laxatives such as Metamucil, is made from the husks of the tiny seeds of the plantago plant (also called plantain). Psyllium seeds, sometimes called fleaseeds, are sold in well-stocked health food stores, sometimes under the slightly misleading name natural vegetable powder. To use psyllium, stir a small amount (about a teaspoon) into an eight-ounce glass of water or juice; drink all the mixture immediately. Results usually occur in twelve to twenty-four hours.

Flaxseed is often suggested as a good fiber source, but these seeds are quite high in natural fat (linseed oil) and could actually worsen your IBS. If you wish to use flaxseed, select a defatted powdered brand.

Slippery elm bark is a useful herbal remedy that acts as

a bowel lubricant. Try stirring two teaspoons of powdered bark into a glass of water or juice.

Peppermint oil is a valuable herbal remedy for relieving painful colon spasms. Enteric-coated capsules, which release the peppermint oil when they reach your intestines, are the best approach. Take one or two capsules three times daily between meals. For mild cramps, strong peppermint tea may be enough. To brew the tea, steep one or two tablespoons of dried peppermint leaves in one cup of boiling water for ten minutes. Sip slowly. Alternatively, add five to ten drops of peppermint oil to a cup of hot water and sip slowly. Other herbs that help relieve spasms include chamomile and valerian. Brew these herbs into strong teas and sip them slowly to relieve mild cramping. Cramping and nausea from gas are sometimes relieved by taking ginger. To make ginger tea, steep one teaspoon of freshly grated or finely chopped fresh ginger in one cup of boiling water for ten minutes. Strain before drinking. Tea bags containing dried ginger can be bought at health food stores; these work almost as well as making your own tea from fresh ginger. Capsules containing dried ground ginger are available at health food stores too. Try taking one 500-milligram capsule instead of a cup of ginger tea. Additional ginger tea or capsules can be taken as needed.

Vitamin and mineral supplements Within the limits of your food sensitivities, try to eat a well-balanced, interesting diet. To be sure you're getting enough vitamins and minerals, take a high-quality multisupplement every day. If you are lactose intolerant and can't have milk or milk products, you may have trouble getting enough calcium in your diet. Since calcium is vital for healthy bones and preventing osteoporosis (especially for menopausal women), you may need to take a supplement to make sure you are getting at least 1,500 milligrams a day.

Other supplements   Rice bran oil, which contains gamma oryzanol, is often helpful for soothing and preventing IBS symptoms. Try taking three 100-milligram capsules daily for four to six weeks; continue if you find it helpful. The amino acid glutamine is vital for fueling and healing your intestinal tract, and it could help relieve IBS. Try taking eight grams a day, in capsules or in powder form mixed with water, for four weeks. Continue if you find it helpful.

Frequent diarrhea or alternating diarrhea and constipation can lead to an imbalance in the bowel microorganisms. If you can tolerate dairy products, try eating six ounces of unflavored live-culture yogurt every day. If not, try taking beneficial bacteria supplements as discussed above in the section on the toxic bowel. Many of our IBS patients find that correcting a bacterial overgrowth helps their symptoms quite a bit.

Juice therapy   Freshly made vegetable juices are a good way to get extra fiber and fluid. Avoid fruit juices, however. The sugar, especially the sorbitol, in fruit juices can cause diarrhea if you have IBS.

Hydrotherapy   The importance of drinking plenty of liquids every day cannot be stressed enough for IBS patients. Drink at least six to eight eight-ounce glasses of pure water daily.

Although activated charcoal in water is a widely used hydrotherapy remedy for gas and diarrhea, do not use it if you have IBS. Activated charcoal could aggravate your symptoms.

Homeopathic remedies   Nux vomica 6c is a homeo-pathic remedy that is particularly helpful for spasms; take every fifteen minutes for up to four doses.

Relaxation techniques   Because stress often brings on or worsens IBS symptoms, any technique that helps you recognize and deal with stress will help. Yoga exercises are quite helpful for many people. Others benefit from learning progressive relaxation techniques. Biofeedback can be extremely effective, especially in combination with counseling on stress reduction. Hypnotherapy is sur-prisingly helpful as well.

Combined Treatments

Diet and stress reduction   If you add fiber to your diet, avoid problem foods, and learn to cope with stress, your irritable bowel syndrome will improve markedly and may even disappear completely for long periods.

ULCERATIVE COLITIS

A disease that causes ulceration and inflammation of the inner lining of the large intestine and rectum, ulcerative colitis causes abdominal pain (especially on the lower left side) and bloody diarrhea. Other symptoms include fatigue, weight loss, loss of appetite, and rectal bleeding. Some 250,000 Americans have ulcerative colitis. It oc-curs mostly in young people ages fifteen to forty, al-though older people sometimes develop the disease too. Ulcerative colitis is usually a chronic, lifelong disease. The cause is unknown, although many researchers be-lieve it is a form of autoimmune disease. Other re-searchers believe that leaky gut syndrome could play a role. There is no cure, but most patients lead normal, productive lives and often have long symptom-free periods. If you have ulcerative colitis, however, your risk of colon cancer is much greater than average.

To diagnose ulcerative colitis, your doctor will take a thorough medical history and do a complete physical examination. In order to detect the inflammation along the bowel lining, you may need to have a barium X ray, also sometimes called a lower GI (gastrointestinal) series or air contrast study. This is an unpleasant, tiring, but necessary procedure in which barium, a chalky substance that is resistant to X rays, is inserted into your colon. The barium lets your doctor see your colon on the X-ray film and check for any obstructions, masses, or defects that could be causing your symptoms. Your colon must be cleansed of all fecal matter for the X ray to be useful, so follow your doctor's instructions carefully to prepare—this is not the sort of test you want to repeat. You will probably be on a clear liquid diet for twenty-four hours before the procedure. You will also probably have to take laxatives and an enema the night before. During the procedure, the barium will be inserted through a nozzle in your rectum and then the X rays will be taken. The barium will cause you to feel abdominal cramps and a powerful urge to defecate. As soon as the X rays have been taken, you will be able to go to the bathroom and eliminate the barium. After that, your colon still has a light coating of barium. Often, but not always, you will then have some additional X rays. This time, air will be pumped into your colon. You will probably feel a sensation like bad gas pains while the air is inside you, but these will stop as soon as the air is expelled.

A barium enema can be a difficult, stressful, and embarrassing experience for you. Remember, however, that the medical staff at the testing center is used to it all—nothing you say, do, or expel will surprise or bother them. Try to relax and keep your sense of humor. After the barium X ray, drink plenty of fluids to avoid constipation. Your doctor may also prescribe a laxative. Your stool will probably be chalky white for a few days afterward from the remaining barium—this is perfectly normal.

Your doctor will also do a sigmoidoscopy and possibly also a colonoscopy to look for inflammation in the lining of your colon and rectum. The sigmoidoscopy lets your doctor look at the last ten to twelve inches of the lower colon and rectum. A narrow, hollow instrument called a sigmoidoscope is inserted gently into the rectum and the area is examined carefully. You may need to take a laxative or enema in advance, and the procedure itself is somewhat uncomfortable. But it usually takes only fifteen or twenty minutes, and you feel fine afterward.

A colonoscopy examines the entire large intestine. The instrument used is a colonoscope, a long, thin, flexible instrument that uses optical fibers to see all the way into your colon. The colonoscope also contains channels that can be used to inflate the colon with air or to take tiny samples of the bowel tissue. Your colon must be cleansed of all fecal matter before the colonoscopy. Follow your doctor's instructions carefully to prepare. You will probably be on a clear liquid diet for forty-eight hours before the procedure. You will also probably have to take laxatives and an enema the night before. During the procedure, you will probably be given a relaxing sedative such a diazepam (Valium) intravenously, although you will be conscious the entire time. You may feel some cramping pains similar to gas pains during the procedure, although in general the procedure is not really painful. In all, a colonoscopy takes about an hour. Because you have been on a liquid diet for two days, you may feel very tired afterward. You can usually go back to your normal diet as soon as the test is over, and most people recover completely in a day or so.

Traditional Treatments

Diet Careful attention to diet is extremely important if you have ulcerative colitis. As with many other bowel problems, dietary fiber is helpful. Avoiding foods that cause flare-ups is also very important. Many people with ulcerative colitis are also lactose intolerant and should avoid all milk and milk products (see the section on lactose intolerance in chapter 5 for more information). Some people with ulcerative colitis are sensitive to grains, particularly wheat and corn, and do much better when these foods are eliminated from the diet. Sugar and artificial sweeteners such as sorbitol may also cause problems. Again, eliminating these foods from your diet could help relieve your symptoms. Spicy foods are also common triggers. Every ulcerative colitis patient is different, however, and has different reactions to specific foods. A simple way to discover which foods you should avoid is to keep a food diary of what you eat and note which foods seem to upset you. Over a period of several weeks, note what you eat at each meal and in between; also note your symptoms. You should soon be able to relate specific foods to specific reactions and thus avoid the foods that cause problems. Be cautious about adding new foods to your diet. Read all food labels carefully to avoid hidden problem foods.

Some ulcerative colitis patients improve markedly when they go on a low-fat diet that eliminates grains, dairy products, sugar, alcohol, chocolate, and some vegetables, including potatoes, soy foods, and chick peas. Meats such as lamb, pork, beef, and poultry are allowed, as are fish and eggs, live-culture yogurt, some cheese, and fresh fruits. Fresh or frozen vegetables are allowed. Butter, lard, and tropical oils such as palm oil should be avoided, although vegetable oils made from corn, olives, safflowers, and sunflowers are acceptable. If you are not lactose intolerant, you can add dairy products to the food list; similarly, grains that are not a problem for you can be added as well. Following this restricted diet for several weeks will probably calm down your symptoms. Continue to follow it for six months, then slowly and cautiously add other safe foods to your diet. Continue to avoid foods to which you are sensitive.

Dietary fiber can help control ulcerative colitis and prevent relapses, but caution is needed. Add fiber slowly to your diet and cut back if you have gas, bloating, or diarrhea. Soluble fiber is very helpful, but insoluble fiber could cause problems for you or even worsen your symptoms if you are having a flare-up. Peel vegetables if possible and always steam them well until they are soft. Avoid raw vegetables. Beans must be thoroughly cooked until they are soft, and even then they may cause problems. Fruit contains large amounts of valuable soluble fiber, including pectin, which is easily digested and can be very helpful for ulcerative colitis. However, even this fiber may be too irritating—you might even have to stew the fruit. Whether you eat fruit raw or cooked, always peel it. Raw fruits should be eaten only if they are fully ripe and soft. Canned fruit in its own natural juice (no sugar added) is a good choice. Cooked breakfast cereals such as oatmeal or cream of wheat are good, easily digestible sources of soluble fiber. Avoid high fiber cold cereals such as bran flakes. In general, avoid rough foods such as popcorn.

If you need a fiber supplement, your doctor will probably recommend one that contains psyllium seeds. These supplements work very well because they form a soft gel in your colon. Don't use any other sort of fiber supplement for ulcerative colitis.

Because ulcerative colitis causes appetite loss, poor absorption of nutrients through the intestines, and frequent diarrhea, you might not be getting enough protein and other nutrients, especially if your diet must be fairly restricted to help prevent flare-ups. It's important to get the best nutrition possible from your diet to compensate. You may find that eating several small meals a day instead of three larger ones can help. Eating nutritious snacks when you are hungry between meals is also helpful—don't fill up on high-calorie, low-nutrition snacks. Discuss liquid meal products such as Ensure with your doctor before you try them.

The severe diarrhea of ulcerative colitis can lead to imbalances in your body's fluids. If you are having diarrhea, be sure to drink plenty of clear fluids such as water, chicken broth, mild herbal teas. Eat soft, bland foods such as rice or oatmeal that you know you can tolerate. Blenderizing your food may help.

If you are having a severe diarrhea attack, call your doctor. You may need to eat nothing but clear fluids for a few days; you may also need medicine to stop the diarrhea. In very severe cases, hospitalization and intravenous feeding may be necessary. In such cases, patients are usually nourished by total parenteral nutrition (TPN). A solution containing protein, fat, and carbohydrates is dripped directly into a large vein (usually in the chest or neck) to provide complete nutrition without absorption through the intestines. TPN is generally used for a few days or weeks until the intestines have healed enough for you to return to a normal diet. In some cases, however, TPN can used be for months or even longer.

Self-help steps   Studies show that the risk of ulcerative colitis in smokers is reduced by 50 percent or more—perhaps the only known example of a beneficial effect from smoking. On the other hand, smokers are twice as likely to develop Crohn's disease, another form of irritable bowel disease that we'll discuss in detail below. If you have ulcerative colitis and you smoke, obviously you're not in the protected group. Stop smoking. If you have ulcerative colitis and you don't smoke, cigarettes are unlikely to help, and they will cause you to have other health problems.

Drugs   The symptoms of ulcerative colitis sometimes need to be controlled with prescription drugs. Inflammation and pain from mild to moderate episodes is often helped by sulfasalazine (Azulfidine), a drug that combines a sulfa preparation with an aspirinlike compound called 5-ASA. Once your symptoms are in remission, you may still have to continue to take the drug to help prevent a recurrence. If your doctor prescribes sulfasalazine, be sure to take the pills with a full glass of water and to drink plenty of liquids during the day. Because sulfasalazine can cause blood problems, you will have to visit your doctor regularly to be checked. This drug may also make your skin more sensitive to sunlight. Some people are allergic to sulfa drugs and should not take sulfasalazine.

Drugs that contain just 5-ASA can also be very helpful.

Mesalamine is the generic name for one form that is inserted into the rectum by a suppository or enema. Mesalamine is particularly helpful if your ulcerative colitis primarily affects your rectum and the lower portion of your colon. The oral form of 5-ASA is known generically as olsalazine. It is taken as a capsule and is most effective if your ulcerative colitis affects the upper portion of your colon. Olsalazine is also helpful for preventing relapses once your colitis is in remission. Drugs containing 5-ASA usually have very few side effects, although a few people are allergic to them.

Steroid drugs such as prednisone may be prescribed if your symptoms are very severe. These drugs must be used with great caution because of their potential side effects. If your doctor prescribes steroids, discuss taking them in the form of an enema, suppository, or topical foam to reduce side effects.

Sometimes the severe diarrhea of ulcerative colitis can be helped with prescription drugs that contain opium or paregoric. Drugs combining diphenoxylate and atropine (Lomotil, Diphenatol, Lomanate, or the generic equivalent) should not be used if you have ulcerative colitis.

Infections, particularly in the lower portion of the colon and the rectum, often complicate ulcerative colitis. Metronidazole (Flagyl) is often prescribed if an antibiotic is necessary.

Interestingly, some ulcerative colitis patients find that wearing a nicotine skin patch relieves their symptoms. If you wish to try this, talk to your doctor first.

Surgery   In about 20 to 25 percent of all cases, the inflammation from ulcerative colitis eventually causes such severe bleeding, scarring, and even perforation that the entire colon and rectum must be removed, a procedure called proctocolectomy. After surgery, an artificial opening called a stoma is created in the abdominal wall. The ileum, or lower portion of the small intestine, is attached to the opening (ileostomy) so that the liquid bowel waste can empty into a bag appliance attached over the stoma. A new surgical technique called a continent ileostomy lets some patients avoid the use of a bag appliance. Another new technique, called ileoanal anastomosis, removes the colon but saves the rectum. The ileum is attached to the rectum so patients can evacuate normally.

Complementary Treatments

Beneficial bacteria supplements   The frequent diarrhea and other problems of ulcerative colitis can cause your colon bacteria to get out of balance. As discussed above in the section on the toxic bowel, a bacterial overgrowth can cause unpleasant symptoms and could make your colitis symptoms worse. Ask your health care provider about doing a comprehensive digestive stool analysis (CDSA). If an imbalance is detected, try using beneficial bacteria as discussed above to correct it.

Herbal therapy   Demulcent herbs that contain mucilage are soothing to the inflamed tissues of your bowel. Licorice root, marshmallow, and slippery elm bark are two common demulcent herbs. You can either use them to brew tea, take them as capsules, or use tinctures mixed with water. These herbs are quite mild. You can safely drink up to four cups a day of the tea.

Licorice root *(Glycyrrhiza glabra)* can be taken as a tea made from a teaspoonful of the licorice root (easily available at health food stores) steeped in half a cup of water for five minutes. Strain before drinking; take half a cup three times a day after meals. We prefer our patients to use deglycyrrhizinated licorice (DGL) in capsules. During attacks, take two or three capsules four times a day. Taking this form is more convenient and is less likely to cause side effects. Licorice root and DGL can cause you to retain fluids. Don't use either if you have high blood pressure, heart disease, liver disease, or diabetes. Stop using licorice root if you notice any swelling in your face, hands, or feet, and don't use it for longer than four weeks.

Marshmallow root is another popular demulcent herb. Combine one teaspoonful of marshmallow root with one cup of water and simmer for fifteen minutes. Let cool and strain before drinking. Take no more than three cups a day after meals.

Another soothing demulcent is slippery elm bark. To make slippery elm bark tea, combine one teaspoon of the bark in two cups of water for twenty minutes. Cool it and strain before drinking. Drink no more than four cups a day. Slippery elm bark is also available in convenient capsules. Take two to four capsules daily.

Goldenseal, an herb that both soothes and helps heal the bowel, may also ease a flare-up of ulcerative colitis. Take two or three capsules four times a day.

Vitamin and mineral supplements   People with ulcerative colitis must be sure they are getting enough vitamins and minerals. At the least, they should take a good daily multivitamin-and-mineral supplement that contains zinc, a mineral that is important for healing. The antioxidant vitamins are extremely important. We suggest taking a total of 10,000 IU mixed carotenes, 500 milligrams vitamin C, and 400 IU vitamin E daily. Drugs such as sulfasalazine can block your body's uptake of B vitamins, so take a complete B formula as well. Be sure it contains folic acid (folate). The B vitamin PABA is sometimes helpful for relieving inflammation for people with ulcerative colitis. Try taking 1,000 to 2,000 milligrams three times daily.

Other supplements   Rice bran oil, which contains gamma oryzanol, is often helpful for soothing and preventing ulcerative colitis symptoms. Try taking three 100-milligram capsules daily for four to six weeks; continue if you find it helpful. The amino acid glutamine is vital for fueling and healing your intestinal tract. Taking eight grams a day, in capsules or in powder form mixed with water, could help relieve the inflammation and help your colon heal. Try glutamine for four to six weeks. Continue if you find it helpful.

Butyric acid, a primary fuel for nourishing the cells lining the colon, is produced by the beneficial bacteria that digest soluble fiber. If you have ulcerative colitis, however, you may not be producing enough butyric acid, especially if you have diarrhea a lot. Butyric acid capsules can help provide the nourishment your colon needs to heal. Try taking three with each meal. Some patients find that retention enemas made from the contents of four to six butyric acid capsules in four ounces of lukewarm water are more effective. Retain the fluid for as long as you can to absorb the butyric acid through the colon wall. Use retention enemas only once a day while you are having a flare-up of symptoms. Do not use them to induce a bowel movement.

Quercetin, an antiinflammatory bioflavonoid, helps relieve pain for some ulcerative colitis patients. Try taking 500 to 1,000 milligrams with meals.

Omega-3 fatty acids, better known as fish oil, are helpful for relieving inflammation. Cold-water fish such as halibut, salmon, mackerel, and tuna are good dietary sources. For relieving ulcerative colitis, however, you will probably need to take fish oil in capsules. These can be bought at health food stores. They are sometimes labeled as EPA (eicosapentanoic) capsules. For fish oil to be effective, however, you will need to take a large dose, up to fifteen capsules a day. As we'll discuss in the section on Crohn's disease below, taking this much fish oil has serious drawbacks, although the newly available enteric-coated capsules are very good.

The omega-3 fatty acids of fish oil are also found in some seaweeds and in carrageenan, an extract made from seaweed. But it is not a good idea to use seaweed products if you have ulcerative colitis—it will make your symptoms worse.

Relaxation techniques The discomfort and embarrassment of an ulcerative colitis flare-up can cause you to feel depressed and anxious, which in turn can worsen the severity of the attack. Try to take it easy, both physically and mentally, during the attack. Relaxation techniques or meditation can help you cope with the pain and break the depressive cycle.

Combined Treatments

Diet and glutamine Careful attention to diet is vital for controlling ulcerative colitis and preventing flare-ups. The amino acid glutamine helps nourish and heal the lining of the colon and could help prevent attacks.

Diet, medication, and herbs If you are having an attack, eat only soft, bland, easily digested foods. Take your medicine as prescribed by your doctor. Demulcent herbs such as licorice root or slippery elm bark may help relieve abdominal pain.

CROHN'S DISEASE

Crohn's disease (also sometimes called ileitis or regional ileitis) is a chronic disorder that causes inflammation or ulceration in the small intestine and often also in the large intestine; in some cases, only the colon is involved. All layers of the intestinal wall, not just the lining, are affected. The inflammation may be found only in patches, but it is quite extensive in severe cases. The symptoms of Crohn's disease can vary widely among patients and often resemble those of other bowel diseases, such as ulcerative colitis or irritable bowel syndrome.

The most common symptoms of Crohn's disease are abdominal pain, often in the lower right part of the abdomen, and diarrhea. Some patients also have rectal bleeding, weight loss, appetite loss, and fever. Sores in the anal area, hemorrhoids, fissures (cracks), and fistulas (abnormal openings from the bowel to the skin surface near the anus) are also symptoms of Crohn's disease.

Although most people with Crohn's disease develop it as children or young adults, the cause is unknown. The disease tends to come and go, with flare-ups and symptom-free periods (often for years), but most people who have Crohn's disease have it all their lives. Relapses are sometimes caused by specific actions, such as eating certain foods, but in most cases, the reason for the relapse is unknown.

At least 500,000 and possibly as many as a million people in the United States have Crohn's disease. The causes remain unknown, although some researchers believe it is a form of autoimmune disease. Both Crohn's disease and ulcerative colitis tend to run in families. In about 15 to 20 percent of all cases, the patient has a close relative who also has inflammatory bowel disease.

Reaching the correct diagnosis in Crohn's disease can take some time and a number of tests. As described above in the section on ulcerative colitis, your physician will take a careful medical history and do a complete physical examination. You will probably also need to have a barium X ray, a sigmoidoscopy, and a colonoscopy.

For more information about living with Crohn's disease and ulcerative colitis, contact:

Crohn's and Colitis Foundation of America
386 Park Avenue South, 17th floor
New York, NY 10016
(800) 343-3637

Traditional Treatments

Diet As with ulcerative colitis, diet is very important for managing Crohn's disease. If you have Crohn's disease, please read the section above on diet for ulcerative colitis—the advice is basically identical. By getting enough dietary fiber, avoiding foods that cause your symptoms to flare up, and eating a nutritious diet, you can be sure of getting adequate nutrition. Again as discussed above in the section on ulcerative colitis, soluble fiber is usually very helpful, although insoluble fiber can cause problems. In general, it is best to eat vegetables that have been peeled and cooked until soft. Peel all fruits.

The food sensitivities connected to ulcerative colitis also play a role in Crohn's disease. Some people with Crohn's disease are also lactose intolerant and find that their symptoms improve markedly when they avoid milk and dairy products. Sugar is also a trigger—if you have

Crohn's disease, avoid sugary foods. Particular foods can also cause flare-ups of Crohn's disease symptoms. Wheat, corn, tomatoes, citrus fruits, eggs, alcohol, and spicy foods are common culprits, although any food may be a problem for a particular patient. Some studies suggest that yeast can also cause symptoms to recur. If you think yeast might be causing problems for you, avoid yeast-raised bread, yogurt, beer, and fermented foods in general.

If you are having diarrhea, be sure to drink plenty of clear fluids such as water, chicken broth, and mild herbal teas. Eat soft, bland foods such a rice or oatmeal that you know you can tolerate. Blenderizing your food may help.

It's particularly important for children with Crohn's disease to get adequate nutrition; otherwise, they may have slowed growth. Sometimes doctors recommend special high-calorie nutritional supplements for children.

Self-help steps Fistulas, fissures, and other painful problems of the rectum are a complication of Crohn's disease. Careful attention to hygiene can help keep the problem under control.

Drugs As with ulcerative colitis, drugs containing 5-ASA, also known as mesalamine, can be very helpful. Mesalamine is generally inserted into the rectum by a suppository or enema. It is particularly helpful if your symptoms are primarily in your rectum and the lower portion of your colon. The oral form of 5-ASA is known generically as olsalazine. It is taken as a capsule and is most effective if your symptoms are in the upper portion of your colon. Olsalazine is also helpful for preventing relapses once your Crohn's disease is in remission. Drugs containing 5-ASA usually have very few side effects, although a few people are allergic to them. Generally speaking, you will need to take the drugs only until your symptoms go into remission.

Steroid drugs such as prednisone may be prescribed if your symptoms are very severe. These drugs must be used with great caution because of their potential side effects. If your doctor prescribes steroids, discuss taking them in the form of an enema, suppository, or topical foam to reduce side effects. You will usually need to take steroids only until your symptoms go into remission.

Sometimes the severe diarrhea of Crohn's disease can be helped with prescription drugs that contain opium or paregoric. However, antidiarrheal drugs combining diphenoxylate and atropine (Lomotil, Diphenatol, Lomanate, or the generic equivalent) should not be used if you have Crohn's disease.

Infections, particularly in the lower portion of the colon and the rectum, often complicate Crohn's disease. Metronidazole (Flagyl) is often prescribed if an antibiotic is necessary. Other antibiotics may be needed to treat rectal problems such as fissures or fistulas.

Recently, researchers have found that the hormone GLP-2 stimulates growth of the lining of the small intestine. Since many people with Crohn's disease have inflammation of the lower portion of the small intestine, it is possible that GLP-2 could help repair the damage and relieve their symptoms. As of now, GLP-2 is not available to patients, but studies are continuing and it is possible that it will be on the market within the next few years.

Surgery In severe cases, surgery to remove diseased portions of the colon may be advised, but this is fairly rare. Surgery is more commonly used in Crohn's disease to treat obstructions of the small or large intestine, abscesses in the bowel, and fistulas in the rectum.

Complementary Treatments

Beneficial bacteria supplements The frequent diarrhea and other problems of Crohn's disease can cause your colon bacteria to get out of balance. As discussed above in the section on the toxic bowel, a bacterial overgrowth can cause unpleasant symptoms and make your colitis symptoms worse. Ask your health care provider about doing a comprehensive digestive stool analysis (CDSA). If an imbalance is detected, use beneficial bacteria as discussed above to try to correct it.

Herbal therapy Demulcent herbs that soothe the intestinal lining can help relieve the pain of Crohn's disease. As discussed above in the section on ulcerative colitis, popular demulcent herbs include marshmallow, slippery elm bark, and licorice root. These mild herbs can be taken either as a tea, by mixing tinctures with water, or in capsules.

If you wish to try licorice root, it may be best to use it in the form of capsules containing deglycyrrhizinated licorice (DGL). Licorice root and DGL can cause you to retain fluids, however, so don't use either if you have high blood pressure, heart disease, liver disease, or diabetes. Stop using licorice root if you notice any swelling in your face, hands, or feet, and don't use it for longer than four weeks.

To use marshmallow root, combine one teaspoonful of marshmallow root with one cup of water and simmer for fifteen minutes. Let cool and strain before drinking. Take no more than three cups a day after meals.

To make slippery elm bark tea, combine one teaspoon

of the bark in two cups of water for twenty minutes. Let cool, then strain before drinking. Drink no more than four cups a day. Slippery elm bark is also available in convenient capsules. Take two to four capsules daily.

Goldenseal, an herb that both soothes and helps heal the bowel, may also be helpful when you have a flare-up of Crohn's disease. Take two or three capsules four times a day.

Vitamin and mineral supplements Because Crohn's disease causes diarrhea and loss of appetite, it's very important to make sure you are getting enough vitamins and minerals. Be sure to take a good daily multivitamin-and-mineral supplement that contains zinc, a mineral that is important for healing. The antioxidant vitamins are also extremely important. We suggest taking 10,000 IU mixed carotenes, 500-milligrams of vitamin C, and 400 IU vitamin E daily. Drugs such as sulfasalazine and mesalamine can block your body's uptake of B vitamins, so take a complete B formula as well. Be sure it contains folic acid (folate). The B vitamin PABA is sometimes helpful for relieving intestinal inflammation. Try taking 1,000 to 2,000 milligrams three times daily.

Other supplements Rice bran oil, which contains gamma oryzanol, is often helpful for soothing intestinal inflammation. Try taking three 100-milligram capsules daily for four to six weeks; continue if you find it helpful. The amino acid glutamine is vital for fueling and healing your intestinal tract. Taking eight grams a day, in capsules or in powder form mixed with water, could help relieve the inflammation and help your colon heal. Try glutamine for four to six weeks. Continue if you find it helpful.

Butyric acid, a primary fuel for nourishing the cells lining the colon, is produced by the beneficial bacteria that digest soluble fiber. If you have Crohn's disease, however, you may not be producing enough butyric acid, especially if you have diarrhea a lot. Butyric acid capsules can help provide the nourishment your colon needs to heal. Try taking three with each meal. Some patients find that retention enemas made from the contents of four to six butyric acid capsules in four ounces of lukewarm water are more effective. Retain the fluid for as long as you can to absorb the butyric acid through the colon wall. Use retention enemas only once a day while you are having a flare-up of symptoms. Do not use them to induce a bowel movement.

Quercetin, an antiinflammatory bioflavonoid, helps relieve pain for some Crohn's patients. Try taking 500 to 1,000 milligrams with meals.

Other supplements Fish oil capsules have been shown to be helpful for reducing flare-ups of Crohn's disease. The EPA component in the fish oil helps to reduce your body's production of leukotrienes, which can help to break the inflammation cycle. Unfortunately, the dose large enough to be helpful (fifteen capsules a day) may also cause you to have gas, nausea, heartburn, and diarrhea. Even worse, it will cause "fish breath" and an unpleasant fishy body odor. A recent European study has shown, however, that time-release fish-oil capsules, which are coated so that the fish oil is not released until it reaches your intestines, have far fewer side effects and virtually eliminate the fishy smell. In the study, the coated capsules were given to patients whose disease was in remission. After a year, 59 percent of the patients were still in remission, compared to 26 percent in a comparison group.

The omega-3 fatty acids of fish oil are also found in some seaweeds and in carrageenan, an extract made from seaweed. Do not use seaweed products if you have Crohn's disease—it will make your symptoms worse.

Juice therapy If you are having a flare-up of Crohn's symptoms, try drinking fresh cantaloupe juice. The beta-carotene and high mineral content of cantaloupe juice, along with its high level of the antioxidant enzyme glutathione, help soothe and heal inflammation in the intestines. Cantaloupe juice may have a laxative effect, however, so start with small amounts. Even if the juice doesn't affect your bowels, drink only a cup or so a day, divided into morning and evening doses.

Relaxation techniques All bowel problems are generally worsened by stress, although stress is not the cause of Crohn's disease. Flare-ups can cause a great deal of discomfort, pain, and embarrassment that lead in turn to depression and anxiety, which in turn worsen the symptoms. In addition, the disruption that a flare-up causes for you and your family, especially if hospitalization is required, can lead to more stress. Try to take it easy, both physically and mentally, during the attack. Relaxation techniques or meditation can help you cope with the pain and break the stress cycle. During remission periods, regularly practicing meditation or relaxation techniques could help prevent a relapse or make the relapse less severe.

Combined Treatments

Diet, glutamine, and fish oil　Careful attention to diet is vital for controlling Crohn's disease and preventing flare-ups. The amino acid glutamine helps nourish and heal the lining of the colon and could help prevent attacks. Fish oil has been shown to help prevent relapses, but it is sometimes difficult to tolerate in the doses required to be helpful.

Diet, medication, and herbs　If you are having an attack, eat only soft, bland, easily digested foods. Take your medicine as prescribed by your doctor. Demulcent herbs such as licorice root or slippery elm may help relieve abdominal pain.

DIVERTICULAR DISEASE

Ideally, the walls of your colon are smooth. Often, however, small, saclike swellings or "pouches" called diverticula (diverticulum in the singular) can develop in the walls of the lowest part and project out into the abdominal cavity. In many cases, the diverticula cause few or no symptoms, a condition called diverticulosis. Sometimes, however, the diverticula become inflamed, causing severe pain on the left side of the abdomen, fever, alternating diarrhea and constipation, nausea, and other symptoms. The inflammation, called diverticulitis, needs prompt medical treatment with antibiotics and possibly even surgery. Diverticulosis is quite common among older adults. By some estimates, about half of all Americans over the age of sixty have diverticulosis; only about 10 percent of them, however, will ever develop diverticulitis symptoms.

Diagnosing an acute episode of diverticulitis is fairly straightforward because the pain is so severe and localized. To be on the safe side, your doctor may order an abdominal X ray to make sure you don't have a perforation of the colon that could lead to a serious abdominal infection (peritonitis). Once your attack has cleared up, your doctor will probably want you to have a barium enema to determine the extent of the diverticula and to make sure you don't have any other colon problem. For a description of the barium enema, see the introductory paragraphs of the section on ulcerative colitis above.

Traditional Treatments

Diet Diverticular disease is common in industrialized nations and almost unheard of in less developed countries. The difference is in the amount of fiber in the diet—the typical American diet is very low in fiber, which leads to small, dry, hard stools that you must strain to pass. The pressure causes outpouchings—diverticula—at weak points in the colon wall, especially where blood vessels enter. When fecal matter becomes caught in the diverticula, infection, or diverticulitis, is the result. At one time, diverticulitis was treated by a low-fiber or liquid diet. Today, most doctors recommend plenty of soft fiber to help cope with a mild to moderate attack. Cook fresh vegetables until they are soft; peel all fruits and eat them only if they are ripe and soft. Cooked whole-grain cereals such as oatmeal are excellent during an attack, but avoid rough uncooked cereals such as bran flakes. The best treatment for diverticulitis is a daily diet containing thirty to forty grams of dietary fiber. A high-fiber diet makes your stool large, soft, and easier to expel, which in turn reduces straining and keeps fecal matter moving through your system quickly.

Fresh fruits and vegetables, beans and legumes, oat or rice bran, and whole-grain breads and cereals are all good sources of fiber. Be sure to drink plenty of liquids as well—six to eight eight-ounce glasses a day. Add fiber to your diet gradually to avoid gas, bloating, and diarrhea. If you have these symptoms, cut back on the amount of fiber or add it more slowly. Ideally, you will have five servings a day of fresh fruits and vegetables and several servings a day of whole grains as well. Even adding a small amount of fiber will help, however. Just one or two apples a day helps many patients.

If you have diverticular disease, most doctors recommend that you avoid nuts, popcorn, and foods with small seeds (raspberries, for instance). Undigested particles can get caught in the diverticula and cause inflammation. Many people with diverticular disease also have trouble with constipation. Your doctor may also suggest that you use a bulk-forming laxative containing psyllium seeds on a regular basis. Do not use any other sort of laxative.

In very severe cases, you might need to be hospitalized on an all-liquid diet until the attack clears up.

Self-help steps   In general, do everything you can to prevent constipation. Regular mild exercise tones the abdominal muscles and helps prevent constipation. Losing weight if you are overweight may help prevent a recurrence of diverticular disease.

Drugs   Powerful antibiotics such as ciprofloxacin (Cipro) are needed to treat diverticulitis. However, these drugs kill not only the bacteria causing the infection but also desirable bacteria in the bowel as well. Try eating several ounces of plain live-culture yogurt every day while you are taking the antibiotic and for a week or so after you finish. This may help restore the favorable bacteria to your bowel.

Surgery In very severe cases, recurring diverticulitis may be treated by surgical removal of the affected portion of the colon.

Complementary Treatments

Reflexology Avoiding constipation is very important if you have diverticulosis. Massaging the large intestine points on the soles of your feet and the palms of your hands may help relieve mild constipation. The large intestine points are located between the arch and the heel, on the inner side of each foot. There are several different points that correspond to the ascending, transverse, descending, and sigmoid colons, but applying steady pressure to the overall area is generally sufficient to provide relief. Two points on each palm correspond to the colon. The first point is about an inch below your fourth finger. The second point, which corresponds more closely with the sigmoid colon, is just above your wrist in line with your third finger. Apply steady pressure by rotating your thumb or a golf ball on the hand points. Repeat as needed.

Beneficial bacteria supplements Diarrhea from both diverticulitis and the antibiotics that are used to treat the infection can cause your colon bacteria to get out of balance. As discussed above in the section on the toxic bowel, a bacterial overgrowth can cause unpleasant symptoms and make your diverticulitis symptoms worse. Ask your health care provider about doing a comprehensive digestive stool analysis. If an imbalance is detected, use beneficial bacteria as discussed above to try to correct it.

Herbal therapy   Demulcent herbs that soothe the intestinal lining can help relieve the pain of diverticulitis, but they should be used only in conjunction with antibiotic therapy, not instead of it. As discussed above in the section on ulcerative colitis, popular demulcent herbs include marshmallow, slippery elm bark, and licorice root. These mild herbs can be taken either as a tea, by mixing tinctures with water, or in capsules. If you wish to try licorice root, it may be best to use it in the form of capsules containing deglycyrrhizinated licorice (DGL). Licorice root and DGL can cause you to retain fluids. Don't use it if you have high blood pressure, heart disease, liver disease, or diabetes. Stop using licorice root if you notice any swelling in your face, hands, or feet, and don't use it for longer than four weeks.

Goldenseal, an herb that both soothes and helps heal the bowel, may also help diverticulitis. Take two or three capsules four times a day.

Herbal remedies for constipation should be used only if they provide fiber—do not use any sort of stimulant laxative if you have diverticulosis or diverticulitis. Unsweetened breakfast cereals that contain large amounts of bran, the fibrous outer coating of grains such as wheat, oats, corn, or rice, are a good approach. These cereals are readily available in health food stores and grocery stores. If you prefer, purchase pure bran and sprinkle a few teaspoons on your regular breakfast cereal. As a bonus, bran, especially rice bran and oat bran, may help reduce your blood cholesterol levels.

Psyllium, the ingredient found in many bulk-forming laxatives such as Metamucil, is made from the husks of the tiny seeds of the plantago plant (also called plantain). Psyllium seeds, sometimes called fleaseeds, are sold in well-stocked health food stores, sometimes under the slightly misleading name of natural vegetable powder. Do not use psyllium in seed form—use only the husks. The seeds could get trapped in the diverticula and cause an infection. To use psyllium husk powder, stir a small amount (about a teaspoon) into an eight-ounce glass of water or juice; drink all the mixture immediately. Results usually occur in twelve to twenty-four hours.

Similarly, if you wish to add fiber with flaxseeds, use defatted powdered seeds. The powder, which is available at health food stores, can be mixed with water or juice and drunk immediately, added to blender drinks, or sprinkled on yogurt or breakfast cereal.

Vitamin and mineral supplements   Take a good multivitamin and mineral daily supplement that contains zinc.

Other supplements   Rice bran oil, which contains gamma oryzanol, is often helpful for soothing intestinal inflammation. Try taking three 100-milligram capsules daily while you have discomfort from diverticulitis. The amino acid glutamine is vital for fueling and healing your intestinal tract. Taking eight grams a day, in capsules or in powder form mixed with water, could help relieve the inflammation and help your colon heal. Take it during the diverticulitis attack and for two weeks after the symptoms have gone away.

Juice therapy   Freshly made juices are an easy way to add fiber to your diet, but only if you use a high-quality juicer that leaves most of the natural fiber in the juice. Vegetable juices of all sorts are good—carrot juice is particularly delicious. Be cautious with fruit juices, however, since they are high in calories. In addition, the sorbitol in apple juice and pear juice could cause diarrhea. Don't mix fruit and vegetable juices.

Combined Treatments

Fiber and antibiotics   For mild to moderate attacks of diverticulitis, take the antibiotics your doctor prescribes. Use up all the pills, even if you are feeling better. Add fiber to your diet to help prevent painful straining during the attack and to help prevent another attack in the future.

APPENDICITIS

Your appendix is a small, wormlike structure found at the junction of the small and large intestines. Anywhere from three to nine inches long, your appendix is filled with lymphatic tissue, but it serves no apparent purpose in your body. If your appendix becomes inflamed or infected, however, you will need an appendectomy (surgical removal of the appendix). Nearly 300,000 people a year in the United States have appendectomies. For unknown reasons, about two thirds of them are women. About two thirds of all appendectomy patients are between the ages of fifteen and forty-four.

Appendicitis almost always develops quickly and with no warning. It usually begins with some mild abdominal discomfort felt near the navel. Over the next few hours, the pain gets much worse, especially in the lower right portion of the abdomen just above the appendix. Your abdomen will probably become hard and very sensitive to pressure; you might also have nausea, vomiting, and a slight fever. You may also become constipated. If this happens, do not take a laxative—it could cause your appendix to burst. A burst appendix will cause peritonitis, a life-threatening infection of the abdominal cavity. Sometimes after several hours the symptoms seem to get suddenly better. This is actually a danger sign in appendicitis: it means your appendix is on the verge of bursting or already has. Get emergency medical attention at once if you have the symptoms of appendicitis.

Traditional Treatments

The only treatment for appendicitis is immediate surgical removal. The diagnosis of appendicitis is generally quite easy to make based on your symptoms, but sometimes you will need blood tests or an abdominal X ray to confirm the diagnosis.

An appendectomy takes place under general anesthesia. It is almost always an uncomplicated procedure, taking under an hour. With modern surgical techniques the incision is very small and inconspicuous, so there is little scarring and your recovery is usually fast and relatively painless. Today most patients are discharged from the hospital within a day or two of the surgery and soon return to their normal activities. You will probably want to take things easy for a week or so after the surgery; you should avoid strenuous activities, jogging, heavy lifting, and the like for several weeks.

Diet Your doctor will recommend a soft diet of easily digested foods for the first few days after your surgery. During this time avoid spicy foods or foods that are likely to cause gas. You will quickly be able to return to your normal diet.

Self-help steps For the first few days after your surgery, bowel movements may cause pain around the incision. Your doctor may suggest using a stool softener containing docusate (Colace or a similar brand), which helps to soften the fecal mass and make it easier to pass.

Drugs Your doctor will probably prescribe oral painkillers for a few days after the surgery to help lessen the discomfort. To prevent infection after the surgery, your doctor will prescribe antibiotics for a week or ten days. These drugs are necessary, but they can have the undesirable side effect of killing both beneficial and harmful bacteria in your intestines. To restore desirable bacteria, eat some plain, live-culture yogurt every day. Since most antibiotics work best when taken on an empty stomach, and because dairy products can interfere with their action, eat several ounces of the yogurt two to three hours after taking each pill.

COLORECTAL CANCER

Today colorectal cancer (cancer of the colon or rectum) is the second most common cause of cancer death in the United States (lung cancer being the first). Every year, about 145,000 Americans will be diagnosed with colorectal cancer; some 55,000 people die of it every year. Most people who get colorectal cancer are over the age of fifty, have a history of colorectal polyps, and eat a high-fat, low-fiber diet. Many also have a family history of colorectal cancer. If you fall into any of these categories, the importance of regular medical checkups cannot be stressed enough. When discovered early enough, colorectal cancer can be treated and often cured.

Colorectal cancer can cause many symptoms. The clearest warning sign is a change in bowel habits. Other common symptoms include diarrhea or constipation, blood in the stool, stools that are narrower than usual, a feeling that the bowel does not empty completely, frequent gas pains, and general stomach discomfort such as bloating or cramps. Weight loss for no known reason and constant tiredness are other common colorectal cancer symptoms. Because the symptoms of colorectal cancer are very similar to other, less serious digestive problems, see your doctor if they persist.

To diagnose colorectal cancer, you may need to have a series of barium X rays of your lower digestive tract (a lower GI series). In addition, you may need to have a colonoscopy. (See the sections on diverticulitis and ulcerative colitis for explanation of these tests.)

Traditional Treatments

Diet   Worldwide, the highest rates of colorectal cancer are in industrialized countries where people eat a high-fat, low-fiber diet. Colorectal cancer rates are far lower in countries such as India and China, where people eat less fat and many more fresh vegetables and whole grains. When people move from countries where colorectal cancer is rare to countries where the cancer is common, they too are more likely to develop the disease as their eating habits change for the worse.

Fiber in the diet may help protect against colorectal cancer in several different ways. Fiber adds bulk to the stool, which may help dilute the concentration of carcinogens from toxins in the environment. Bulk also makes the stool pass through your system more quickly, which lessens the amount of time that any carcinogens

are in contact with colon. Fiber may also bind some carcinogens and remove them quickly from your system.
Fiber also works to counteract some of the possibly
harmful effects of fat in the diet. Dietary fat causes you
to produce more bile acids in order to digest them, and
the bile acids and their breakdown products may be carcinogenic in the colon. Dietary fiber may bind some bile
acids and minimize their contact with the colon; by
speeding the transit time of your stool, dietary fiber also
minimizes the amount of time bile acids spend in your
colon.

If you are at risk for colorectal cancer, please read the
section on dietary fiber in chapter 8. For maximum pro-
tection, the first step is to reduce your fat intake, especially fat from processed foods such as sausage and from
red meat. The most important step is to add fresh fruits,
fresh vegetables, and whole grains to your diet. For reasons that are not entirely clear, wheat bran is particularly
helpful. Cruciferous vegetables such as broccoli, cauliflower, and cabbage have plenty of dietary fiber as well
as valuable cancer-fighting phytochemicals and antioxidant vitamins.

People who have two or more alcoholic drinks a day
have higher rates of colorectal cancer. Beer drinkers are
most at risk.

Self-help steps   Regular medical checkups will help
detect colorectal polyps that could become cancerous and
will also detect colorectal cancer in the early stages when
it is most curable. During your checkup, the doctor will
perform a digital rectal exam by inserting a lubricated,
gloved finger into your rectum and feeling for abnormal
areas. If you are age fifty or over, your doctor will also
check for fecal occult (hidden) blood with a painless test.

The presence of blood in the stool could indicate colorectal cancer, although there are many other possible causes. Doctors also recommend a sigmoidoscopy every three to five years if you are over age fifty. In this procedure, the doctor examines your rectum and lower colon with a thin, lighted tube to check for polyps, tumors, and other abnormalities.

If you have a family history of colorectal cancer or are at greater risk for some other reason, your doctor may recommend more frequent checkups and tests.

Surgery A colorectal polyp is a tumor that grows inward from the wall of the colon or rectum. Even benign (noncancerous) colorectal polyps should be removed because they can *become* cancerous. In many cases, your doctor can remove the polyp through a sigmoidoscope, right in the office. The polyp is sent to a lab for biopsy (examination for cancer cells); although in most cases, polyps are benign, a biopsy is the only way to know for sure. If you have had a colorectal polyp, you are likely to develop new ones, so be sure to have regular follow-up exams.

If you are diagnosed with colon cancer, your doctor will order additional tests to learn the extent, or staging, of the disease. Your treatment decisions will depend on the results. Surgery is the most common treatment for colorectal cancer. The type of operation depends on the location and size of the tumor. Most patients have a colectomy. The surgeon removes the part of the colon or rectum that contains the cancer and reconnects the healthy sections. Colectomy is often the only treatment needed for early colorectal cancer.

When the cancer has moved beyond the early stages, the healthy sections sometimes can't be reconnected after the colectomy. In these cases, the surgeon performs a colostomy, creating an opening (stoma) in the abdomen through which solid waste leaves the body, where it is collected in a removable bag. A colostomy may be temporary or permanent. If the cancer is in the rectum, the colostomy will probably be permanent. Only about 15 percent of all colorectal patients need a permanent colostomy.

In some cases, surgery is followed by chemotherapy, to try to prevent the disease from spreading (metastasizing) to other parts of your body. Radiation therapy is sometimes used before surgery to reduce the size of the tumor. It is also sometimes used after surgery to destroy any cancer cells that may still be in the area.

Alternative Treatments

There are no acceptable alternative treatments for colorectal cancer. Treatments such as colonic irrigation, megavitamin therapy, and other alternative (and sometimes fraudulent) practices will not help colorectal cancer. Indeed, the delay in getting needed surgical treatment could allow the cancer to grow larger and spread to other parts of your body.

CHAPTER 10

Hemorrhoids

The pain, itching, burning, swelling, and discomfort of hemorrhoids (also called piles) are experienced by some 25 million Americans. Hemorrhoids, which can be internal or external, occur when the veins in the lower rectum, at the junction with the anal canal, become swollen and bulge out beneath the thin layer of tissue that covers them. Internal hemorrhoids occur in the upper portion of the anal canal and may cause pain, burning, itching, or aching in the area. These hemorrhoids may also bleed, leaving bright red blood on the stool or on the toilet paper after a movement. Internal hemorrhoids are most likely to be troublesome to the point of needing medical attention for pain and bleeding. External hemorrhoids occur under the surface of the skin at the anal opening. They tend to disappear after a few days, but they usually then come back. External hemorrhoids produce pain, swelling, burning, and itching of the overlying skin. Sometimes a painful blood clot (thrombosis) forms in the vein. Many people have mixed internal and external hemorrhoids, a combination of hemorrhoids that looks a little like a cluster of grapes.

A low-fiber diet is almost always the cause of hemorrhoids. Constipation or straining during a bowel movement puts pressure on the network of delicate hemorrhoidal veins, which can cause them to swell and bulge. Lack of exercise, sitting or standing for long periods, being overweight, or doing a lot of lifting are other contributing factors. Often a pregnant woman develops hemorrhoids because of the weight and pressure of the growing baby. These hemorrhoids usually go away after the baby is born.

The symptoms of more serious problems, including fissures, fistulas, inflammatory bowel diseases, and tumors, can be mistaken for the symptoms of hemorrhoids instead. If you have severe pain, seepage, bleeding, protrusion, prolapse, a lump, or thrombosis in the anorectal area, or if you have a change in your bowel habits, see your doctor promptly.

In most cases, uncomfortable hemorrhoid symptoms respond well to self-help steps—particularly, for instance, to adding fiber to the diet. If your hemorrhoids are very painful or if an internal hemorrhoid starts to bleed, see your doctor at once. Prompt medical attention will help keep the problem under control.

An anal fissure is a small, elongated tear or ulcer in the mucous membrane of the anus. The fissure can cause the muscles around the anus to go into spasms, which causes severe pain. In most respects, anal fissures are treated very much as hemorrhoids are. In particular, dietary fiber is very helpful. The goal is to produce a large, soft stool that is easily passed. Once you're no longer straining to pass hard stools, the fissure has a chance to heal—and you'll be less likely to get another one.

While you're healing, try to avoid anything that will give you diarrhea, since this will irritate the fissure further. You might also want to avoid spicy foods and very coarse foods such as nuts or popcorn during this time. To avoid irritating the fissure, your doctor may suggest using a bulk-forming laxative containing psyllium husks; a stool softener such as docusate may also be suggested. An anal fissure can be very painful, so you may have to take it easy for a few days. Warm sitz baths are especially helpful for fissures.

Sometimes a fissure just won't go away, or else it recurs. In either case, your doctor may suggest a minor surgical procedure to remove the fissure. You may have to stay in the hospital for a day or two, but healing is usually very rapid and you can quickly return to your normal activities.

Traditional Treatments

Diet Dietary fiber is essential for treating hemorrhoids and preventing them from getting worse. Fiber in the diet makes your stool bulky, soft, and easy to pass, which reduces straining when you have a bowel movement. To relieve your hemorrhoid symptoms, you should gradually increase your daily fiber intake to at least forty grams a day. You can do this easily by eating two to four servings of fruit, three to five servings of vegetables, and three to four servings of whole grains such as whole wheat bread, oatmeal, or bran cereal. Add fiber to your diet gradually—suddenly adding a lot can lead to bloating, gassiness, diarrhea, and other problems. We've discussed the importance of dietary fiber and ways to prevent constipation at length in chapter 8; if you have hemorrhoids, please read that section carefully.

Drinking plenty of liquids is another easy step toward eliminating constipation. Drink at least six to eight eight-ounce glasses of water or other liquids a day.

An episode of hemorrhoid pain can make bowel movements very painful. This in turn makes you avoid having movements, which causes constipation, which makes bowel movements more painful and worsens your hemorrhoids. At such times, using a bulk-forming laxative or a stool softener may be more helpful than adding dietary fiber. Bulk-forming laxatives contain powdered natural or synthetic fiber. Also sometimes called vegetable or natural laxatives, bulk-forming laxatives absorb water and form a soft gel in your colon, which helps your stool pass easily. Always take bulk-forming laxatives with a full eight-ounce glass of water, fruit juice, or other fluid. Be sure to stir the mixture well and drink it all immediately. Bulk-forming laxatives can be used safely over long periods of time. Emollient laxatives, also known as stool softeners, usually contain docusate, which helps to soften the fecal mass and make it easier to pass. Use emollient laxatives only for short-term treatment; don't take them for longer than a week.

Some people find that particular foods, such as coffee, chocolate, alcohol, or nuts, aggravate their hemorrhoids; very spicy foods or foods with a lot of ginger can also cause problems. Needless to say, if you notice that something you eat or drink makes your hemorrhoids worse, avoid it.

Self-help steps   Careful attention to personal hygiene is important if you have hemorrhoids. Use soft toilet tissue to avoid irritating the inflamed tissue around your anus. Avoid scented or colored bathroom tissue. Cleanse the anal area gently but thoroughly after a bowel movement. You can do this easily with wet, soft toilet tissue or a washcloth and mild soap. Convenient cleansing pads or premoistened wipes (Tucks and similar products) can be purchased in any pharmacy. If you are having a flare-up of hemorrhoid trouble, sitting may be very uncomfortable. Doughnut-shaped cushions or inflatable rings, available at pharmacies and surgical supply stores, can help relieve the discomfort. Getting regular, gentle exercise is often helpful for preventing constipation and toning the abdominal muscles. Avoid lifting heavy objects, however. If you are having a painful flare-up, take it easy and try to stay off your feet and in bed for a day or two. Most flare-ups last for only a few days.

Drugs Many nonprescription products help relieve hemorrhoid symptoms. In general, these products are meant for external use only. Read the labels carefully. For best results, apply hemorrhoid products after, not before, bowel movements. Cleanse and dry the anal area thoroughly before applying the product sparingly. Use a finger to apply a thin film of these products to the anal area and the lower anal canal. To apply these products within the rectum, use a finger, the applicator supplied with the product, or a pile pipe. (Your doctor or pharmacist can explain the use of applicators and pile pipes to you.)

Suppositories are less effective as an application method. If you do use a suppository, be sure to unwrap it before insertion. If a rectal suppository becomes too warm, it will soften and be difficult to insert; store suppositories in a cool place, preferably the refrigerator. Hold softened suppositories under cold running water or place them in the refrigerator to harden them. Do not use a suppository if insertion causes pain.

Protectants reduce irritation, itching, and burning in the anal area by forming a barrier on the skin. The safest, simplest, most effective, and least expensive protectant is plain petroleum jelly (Vaseline or the generic equivalent).

Other popular protectants include mineral oil, shark liver oil, cod liver oil, cocoa butter, and vegetable oil. Do not use lanolin, glycerin, or propylene glycol. Preparation H, a well-known over-the-counter protectant, contains shark liver oil.

Local (topical) anesthetics temporarily help deaden burning, pain, itching, and irritation. These products should be used in the anal region and lower anal canal only. Most products contain benzocaine or pramoxine hydrochloride in an ointment base (Nupercainal, Tronolane, and similar products). Products containing camphor or phenol are not effective and have been taken off the market.

Astringents such as zinc oxide (Anusol, Nupercainal, and similar products) can help relieve itching, burning, and swelling particularly from external hemorrhoids. They should be used externally only.

Some nonprescription hemorrhoid products contain boric acid or resorcinol, which are said to be external antiseptics that can help prevent infection. There is no real evidence to show that these products are any more effective than good hygiene with soap and water.

In severe cases, your doctor will prescribe suppositories or injections containing corticosteroids and pain-killing drugs to shrink the swelling and relieve pain.

Surgery   Although most hemorrhoids heal on their own in a week or two, they sometimes come back, especially if you don't eat more fiber. Sometimes bleeding or other symptoms are so severe that the hemorrhoid must be medically or surgically treated.

Small external hemorrhoids that are causing serious pain can be treated in the doctor's office, with minor surgery to remove the blood clot that has formed and is causing the pain. Painful or bleeding internal hemorrhoids can often be treated by injecting a shrinking medication into the tissue surrounding the hemorrhoid.

More serious internal hemorrhoids are sometimes treated with rubber band ligation. A small rubber band is placed around the base of the hemorrhoid to cut off the flow of blood to the area; the hemorrhoid withers away in about a week. The advantage of this approach is that anesthesia is not needed, and it causes little or no discomfort. Internal hemorrhoids can also be destroyed by burning them away with laser surgery, or freezing them off (cryosurgery). Be wary of clinics that advertise their laser surgery methods; get a second opinion before you proceed with surgery that may be unnecessary.

In the most serious cases, a hemorrhoidectomy may be needed. Your troublesome hemorrhoids will be surgically removed while you are under general anesthesia. You may need to stay in the hospital for a few days, but you can soon return to your normal activities.

Complementary Treatments

Reflexology Massaging the large intestine points on your feet may help relieve hemorrhoid discomfort. The large intestine points are located on the sole between the arch and the heel, on the inner side of each foot. There are several different points that correspond to the ascending, transverse, descending, and sigmoid colons, but applying steady pressure to the overall area is generally sufficient to provide relief. Two points on each palm correspond to the colon. The first point is about an inch below your fourth finger. The second point, which corresponds more closely with the sigmoid colon, is just above your wrist in line with your third finger. Apply steady pressure by rotating your thumb or a golf ball on the hand points. Repeat as needed.

Herbal remedies A number of herbal remedies are helpful for hemorrhoids. Witch hazel (hamamelis water) is a popular astringent treatment for external use only. Purchase only nondistilled witch hazel extract. Distilled witch hazel contains mostly alcohol and is not as effective. If you can't find nondistilled witch hazel extract at your pharmacy, check your health food store. Use a compress to apply witch hazel to the anal area. Moisten a large cotton ball with the witch hazel and hold it against the anal area for five to ten minutes; repeat twice or three times a day.

A European herbal treatment that is becoming popular in the United States is butcher's broom, in ointment or suppository form. This herb contains compounds that help constrict swollen blood vessels and may also have anti-inflammatory properties. Ointments and suppositories containing butcher's broom are now available in the United States at health food stores. Some herbalists also recommend taking 100 milligrams of butcher's broom extract orally three times a day to strengthen blood vessels and improve the circulation. Another European herbal remedy that is often helpful is an oil made from Saint-John's-wort. Salves containing this reddish oil can be purchased in health food stores.

Salves, creams or ointments containing vitamin E, calendula, comfrey, or goldenseal are often helpful. Spread a thin layer of the mixture gently over the anal area.

Vitamin and mineral supplements Vitamin E helps heal inflamed and damaged tissues; take 400 to 800 IU daily during a flare-up. To help build up the strength of your blood vessels and keep them elastic, you need vitamin C and bioflavonoids. Taking 500 to 1,500 milligrams of vitamin C every day may help. Bioflavonoids are found in berries and cherries, but to be sure you're getting enough, take a 500-milligram supplement daily. As a bonus, bioflavonoids may help protect your eyesight from problems such as macular degeneration.

Hydrotherapy Sitz baths or warm compresses can be very helpful and are often recommended by physicians. To take a sitz bath, fill the tub to the depth of three or four inches with warm (not hot) water. Sit in it for ten minutes or so several times a day. Some patients find that adding a quarter cup of Epsom salts to the water has a helpful astringent effect.

Warm compresses can be made by soaking a clean cloth (a washcloth is good) in plain warm (not hot) water and applying it to the anal area. Hold the cloth in place for five to ten minutes; repeat several times a day. A cold compress made by soaking a clean cloth in cold, strong black tea is also often helpful. Hold the compress in place for five to ten minutes; repeat three or four times a day.

Homeopathy Several different oral homeopathic remedies are suggested for hemorrhoids. Hamamelis 6c is recommended if you feel bruised and sore. Sepia 6c is recommended if you have the sensation of a ball in the rectum. Sulphur 6c is recommended if you are having burning and itching. Try these three or four times a day for up to four days. You could also try hamamelis ointment on the rectal area twice a day.

Combined Treatments

Diet, petroleum jelly, and hydrotherapy   Adding
fiber to the diet to prevent constipation and straining is
vital for relieving hemorrhoid discomfort. Petroleum
jelly is a soothing ointment that helps relieve itching. Sitz
baths and warm compresses also are helpful for relieving
swelling and pain during flare-ups.

Glossary

Antacid A substance such as magnesium hydroxide that absorbs excess acid in the stomach.

Antiemetic A substance that helps relieve nausea and prevent vomiting.

Bile A greenish-brown digestive fluid made by the liver. Bile contains cholesterol, bile acids, lecithin, and water; it breaks up and digests fats in the intestines.

Butyric Acid The primary fuel for the cells lining the colon. It is produced by friendly bacteria as they digest fiber in the colon.

Carminative Any herb such as peppermint that relieves gas pain and abdominal cramps by relaxing the muscles of the stomach and intestines.

CDSA See **Comprehensive digestive stool analysis**.

Celiac Disease The inborn inability to digest gluten.

Cholagogue An herb such as dandelion that stimulates the gallbladder to contract, which improves the flow of bile.

Cholecystectomy Surgical removal of the gallbladder.

Choleretic An herb such as dandelion that stimulates the liver to produce bile.

Chyme The soupy mixture of food and digestive juices that leaves your stomach and enters the small intestine.

Colitis General term for inflammation of the colon. See also **Irritable bowel syndrome**.

Colostomy An opening (stoma) in the abdomen through which solid waste leaves the body and is collected in a removable bag.

Comprehensive Digestive Stool Analysis (CDSA) A lab test that analyzes a stool sample for the presence of bacteria, parasites, and other indicators of digestive problems.

Constipation Infrequent or difficult passing of stools.

Crohn's disease An inflammatory disease of the ileum (see **Ileum**) and colon.

Demulcent An herb such as marshmallow, which can be used to sooth the mucous membranes of the digestive tract.

Diarrhea Frequent passing of loose, watery stools.

Duodenal Ulcer A painful, craterlike sore in the mucous membrane lining the duodenum. See **Gastric ulcers; Peptic ulcers.**

Duodenum The first portion of the small intestine.

Dysbiosis Bacterial overgrowth of the small intestine.

Fiber The indigestible portion of plant foods. See also **Soluble fiber; Insoluble fiber.**

Flatulence Intestinal gas.

Fructooligosacchrides (FOS) A dietary supplement that nourishes beneficial bacteria in the intestines.

Gamma Oryzanol A compound found in rice bran oil; useful for its healing effect on the digestive system.

Gastric Ulcer A painful, craterlike sore in the mucous membrane lining your stomach.

Gastritis Inflammation of the mucous membrane lining the stomach.

Gastroenteritis A minor illness affecting the stomach and causing nausea, vomiting, and diarrhea.

Glutamine Amino acid essential for nourishing the cells lining the small intestine.

H₂ Blocker A drug that sharply reduces stomach acid production by blocking the effects of histamine.

Heartburn Painful burning sensation in the upper abdomen caused when stomach acid is forced up into the esophagus.

Helicobacter Pylori The bacterium that causes peptic ulcers.

Hypochlorhydria Too little hydrochloric acid in the stomach.

IBD See **Inflammatory bowel disease.**

IBS See **Irritable bowel syndrome.**

Ileitis Inflammation of the ileum. See also **Crohn's disease.**

Ileum The lower portion of the small intestine.

Inflammatory Bowel Disease (IBD) A disease such as ulcerative colitis or Crohn's disease, which causes inflammation of the lining of the colon.

Insoluble Fiber Dietary fiber consisting primarily of cellulose from the walls of plant cells; it absorbs water in the intestines.

Irritable Bowel Syndrome (IBS) Overall term for a group of symptoms, including crampy pain, gassiness, bloating, diarrhea, constipation, mucus in the stool, and changes in bowel habits—when these are not caused by inflammation in the bowel.

Lactobacilli Friendly bacteria found in the small intestine and colon.

Laxative Substance that stimulates a bowel movement.

Leaky Gut Syndrome Damage to the villi (see **Villi**) of the small intestine that allows undigested food particles to enter the bloodstream.

Nausea Sensation of queasiness or being on the verge of vomiting.

Peptic Ulcer A painful, craterlike sore in the mucous membrane that lines the stomach or the duodenum. Peptic ulcers in the stomach are called gastric ulcers; peptic ulcers in the duodenum are called duodenal ulcers.

Peristalsis Involuntary, wavelike contractions that propel food through the intestines.

Psyllium Seeds of the plantago (plantain) plant; a natural source of fiber found in many bulk-forming laxatives.

Silymarin Liver-protecting compound found in the milk thistle plant.

Soluble Fiber Dietary fiber consisting primarily of pectin, along with mucilage, plant gums, and hemicellulose; it forms a gel in the intestines.

Sprue See **Celiac disease.**

Ulcer See **Peptic ulcer.**

Villi Tiny, fingerlike projections that line the small intestine and increase the area for the absorption of nutrients.

Index

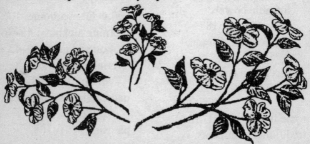